Cambridge Elements ≡

Elements in Histories of Emotions and the Senses
edited by
Rob Boddice
Tampere University
Piroska Nagy
Université du Québec à Montréal (UQAM)
Mark Smith
University of South Carolina

UNCERTAINTY AND EMOTION IN THE 1900 SYDNEY PLAGUE

Philippa Nicole Barr
Australian National University

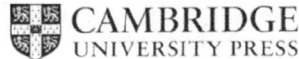

CAMBRIDGE
UNIVERSITY PRESS

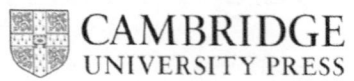

CAMBRIDGE
UNIVERSITY PRESS

Shaftesbury Road, Cambridge CB2 8EA, United Kingdom

One Liberty Plaza, 20th Floor, New York, NY 10006, USA

477 Williamstown Road, Port Melbourne, VIC 3207, Australia

314–321, 3rd Floor, Plot 3, Splendor Forum, Jasola District Centre,
New Delhi – 110025, India

103 Penang Road, #05–06/07, Visioncrest Commercial, Singapore 238467

Cambridge University Press is part of Cambridge University Press & Assessment,
a department of the University of Cambridge.

We share the University's mission to contribute to society through the pursuit ⟨
education, learning and research at the highest international levels of excellen⟨

www.cambridge.org
Information on this title: www.cambridge.org/9781009462105

DOI: 10.1017/9781108908061

First published 2024

A catalogue record for this publication is available from the British Library

ISBN 978-1-009-46210-5 Hardback
ISBN 978-1-108-82106-3 Paperback
ISSN 2632-1068 (online)
ISSN 2632-105X (print)

Uncertainty and Emotion in the 1900 Sydney Plague

Elements in Histories of Emotions and the Senses

DOI: 10.1017/9781108908061
First published online: February 2024

Philippa Nicole Barr
Australian National University

Author for correspondence: Philippa Nicole Barr, philippa.barr@outlook.com

Abstract: When the third global plague pandemic reached Sydney in 1900, theories regarding the ecology and biology of disease transmission were transforming. Changing understandings led to conflicts over the appropriate response. Medical and government authorities employed symbols like dirt to address gaps in knowledge. They used these symbols strategically to compel emotional responses and to advocate for specific political and social interventions, authorising institutional actions to shape social identity and the city in preparation for Australia's 1901 Federation. Through theoretical and historical analysis, this Element argues that disgust and aversion were effectively mobilised to legitimise these actions. As an intervention in contemporary debates about the impact of knowledge on emotion and affect, it presents a case for the plasticity of emotions like disgust, and for how both emotion and affect can change with new medical information.

This Element also has a video abstract: www.cambridge.org/barr

Keywords: disgust, history of emotions and the senses, pandemic disease, history and philosophy of science, cities

ISBNs: 9781009462105 (HB), 9781108821063 (PB), 9781108908061 (OC)
ISSNs: 2632-1068 (online), 2632-105X (print)

Contents

1 Introduction

I signed the contract on this Element in December 2019[*] – only months before the Covid-19 pandemic was declared a worldwide health emergency. As I slowly began working on the draft, I often fielded questions about parallels between the pandemic I was living and the one I was researching. While I noticed certain emotional arcs which were comparable with the historical event that is my focus, I became at least as interested in their differences. Covid-19 is contagious and airborne. It is a viral infection, not bacterial, with a different biology and ability to spread and replicate. But I could see consistencies with the period of transition in medical knowledge at the end of the nineteenth century, as people struggled to understand this disease and how it would affect them. Without everyone agreeing on or knowing everything, amidst the models and theories, how did people's emotions and fears shape their response to plague? How were institutional responses influenced by both medical information and cultural reactions? How did these emotional and affective responses further compel intervention and perception? And how could these questions be historicised? I was interested in how disgust influenced the way people interacted with their environments and one another in Sydney in 1900. How they saw themselves in relation to others, the many others both within and outside themselves. How they imagined themselves in relation to disease at a moment of scientific discovery of bacteria and changing understanding of disease causation.

These questions affected me on a far more personal level while I was working on this manuscript. A few months before the revisions were due back to the publisher, I was diagnosed with a disease caused by bacteria from the same genus as plague, *Yersinia enterocolitica*. The Yersinia genus, I quickly discovered, included *Yersinia pestis*. Like my research subjects, I had experienced Yersinosis. 'At least it is on brand,' I said to a medical historian friend. I even had to take the same antibiotics that are prescribed to people exposed to plague or anthrax today. It was such a relief to have a diagnosis, an agent, an object causing my illness. To know what was wrong. But then it did not get better. I was diagnosed with a secondary infection called Aeromonas and had to undergo more tests. As I worked on this Element, I continued to lose weight and experience other symptoms. And the inflammation, confusion, anxiety, and disgust all got the better of me.

Illness disrupts taken-for-granted ways of doing things. It is a limit situation. Thomas Fuchs describes a 'limit situation' as a moment of 'existential vulnerability, when the fragility of the body becomes recognisable, cognisant

---

[*] This published work is the revised version of a research project originally completed at Macquarie University. The author is currently working at Australian National University (philippa.barr@anu.edu.au) and Western Sydney University (p.barr@westernsydney.edu.au).

(Fuchs 2013, 301). It prevents you from doing things the way you did before. You have to change your ways. Your social relations. It disrupts the way you interpret the world, your sense of safety, of threat, of comfort. It also disrupts the way people interact with you. 'They are like a wall that we run up against, against which we fail' (Fuchs 2013, 303). When I first started sharing my diagnosis some people laughed about it, others were apprehensive. 'But do you have the plague?' some friends asked worriedly when I invited them over for dinner. While I put some fears at ease, others were more apprehensive. I noted that the scientists and medical professionals among my friends or extended family were decidedly more relaxed about the risk to themselves. They had seen this kind of thing before. Experience provided emotional relief even without certainty.

This study of Sydney in 1900 argues that certainty has its limits, and that uncertainty produces emotional responses. This argument is particularly relevant to the early stages of pandemic, but can resonate at other times, in other crises. Different stages of a pandemic entail different work, investigating the cause, charting the course, preventing the spread, looking for a cure or a vaccine. They also provoke different emotions and specific affects. When we do not know what is happening our emotions have more power over us. They compel us. I intend that this Element will be useful for thinking about how emotions colour our response to disease more generally. My approach is to examine the plasticity of disgust in mediating between antibiotic and probiotic worlds, different knowledges and priorities, and in regulating relations in the first outbreak of the plague in Sydney. I explore these issues and justify my decision to use both the emotion and affect of disgust in this Element. It is also a useful investigation into the specificities of disgust and its role in warding off disease.

1.1 Sydney 1900

Sydney had been first settled in 1788 as a colony of the British Empire. But 1900 was its final year as a colony. The city of Sydney and the state of New South Wales were preparing to join with the other Australian colonies in a Federation. These preparations were disrupted and perhaps accelerated by an event: the plague spreading around ports of the British Empire from Hong Kong and reaching Sydney. In China and India millions of people died. Yet the actual number of infections and mortalities from plague were low in Sydney compared to other diseases in the nineteenth century (Curson 1985, 91). Between the 19th of January and the 9th of August 1900, 303 people in Sydney contracted the bubonic plague; 103 died (Ashburton-Thompson 1900b, 8). The 1900 outbreak was the first of a series of ten outbreaks in Sydney that lasted until 1910 and then reappeared in 1921 (Echenberg 2007, 266). Over the course of these 21 years the plague infected more than 1,360 people, of which more than 600 people were in Sydney (Curson 1985, 137). The first outbreak of the plague in Sydney compelled by far the strongest emotion and subsequent reaction of any nineteenth-century epidemic (New South Wales Parliament 1900a, 114).[1]

In New South Wales, as opposed to the other British colonies, the public health response was widely, if not uniformly, supported by the public, who accepted its coercive elements, such as quarantine, lockdowns, and the demolition of homes (Ashburton-Thompson 1907b, 1104). Sydney went into overdrive to distinguish itself from the other cities of empire. As Ashburton-Thompson reflected years later, at the time of the first plague outbreak 'the population of about 500,000 was wholly white, wholly civilised, spoke the mother-tongue of the observers, and had been well trained in obedience to the peremptory discipline of the health authority in the course of several epidemics of smallpox which had been summarily suppressed during the preceding 20 years' (Ashburton-Thompson 1907b, 1104). But while the dream of the colonial cities was one of pure air, wide streets, and clean water, the reality was often fouler than residents, perhaps overly anxious about their colonial status, cared to admit.

The reaction to the 1900 plague was a strong basis of support for the institution of public health which in the case of Sydney was particularly influenced by the new science of bacteriology and the use of epidemiological methods to understand the genesis of disease. These feelings of disgust and fear were instrumentalised to create a kind of social and historical distance, to produce a new identity that was to be part of the Federation of Australia but also independent from the other colonies of empire, those which suffered far greater misfortune in the plague's spread. This identity was marked by negation; not dirty, not diseased, not irresponsible.

In this Element I argue that in Sydney in 1900 there was evidence of the strategic mobilisation of the symbolism of dirt in discourse to channel and produce the response of disgust to advocate for specific political solutions. Actions such as fumigating the city sewers or demolishing properties did not always have their basis in confident public health strategy and were often reactive, aiming to manage the emotions of the public rather than the public health. In the concluding discussion I consider the extent to which our aversion

---

[1] While the 1881 smallpox outbreak also provoked a strong emotional reaction from the public and is certainly interesting for other reasons such as the public reaction to vaccination, it was not equal in force to the response or interventions provoked by the 1900 plague. As Governor William Lyne admonished in a speech to parliament in June 1900, '[t]he small-pox scare was not to be compared to what has taken place of late' (New South Wales Parliament 1900a, 114).

of certain smells or sights helps us to avoid pathogenic bacteria and whether that has in fact shaped the response itself. I therefore tend to side with the symbolic anthropologists like Mary Douglas in considering the properties of dirt from more of a symbolic than a biological perspective. This is not to deny a potentially threatening biological reality to exhaled air or discarded excrement. Indeed, these symbols derive some of their potency from their sensory properties and the ways they may challenge or compromise our complicated biologies.

1.2 The Feeling of Dirt

In public discourse, uncertainty and heightened emotion were resolved using sensory symbols – like bad odours, dirty homes, and threatening bodies. For example, in his thirty-five directions for the management of the epidemic plague at Sydney, Ashburton-Thompson specified the need for local authorities to remember their powers and duties under the Public Health Act and the Municipalities Act, who 'were exhorted to use great exertions to get rid of all accumulations of filth and of nuisances in general' (Ashburton-Thompson 1900b, 18). Like Ashburton-Thompson many politicians, journalists, and con-cerned citizens used terms like 'filth' to empower their ideas for what was happening and why it needed to change. The question is, why was this so effective?

Dirt will always arise in moments of social disruption and confusion. For Douglas, as cultures strive to produce order, or unify an 'inherently untidy' experience, they will inevitably produce dirt (Douglas 1966, 4). Over time, she argues, our efforts to produce order become habits, classifications, and prac-tices. Insofar as these cultures work then we learn to trust them (Douglas 1966, 36–7). Yet there will always be anomalies or ambiguities, compound substances or intermediate states, borderline cases that violate order and provoke a response. To maintain trust, cultures need to continually process ambiguity and anomaly, to clean and create order. Nothing is essentially dirty, but it becomes dirt because it is in the wrong place, on the wrong surface, because it is standing in the wrong position relative to other things. The rubbish on the ground or the Bible kissed by the quarantine contact violates order (Douglas 1966, 2). They simply should not be there. But they cannot exist without relating to something else, a foundation, an object, a space (Enzensberger 1972, 10). Dirt is not a perfect abstract concept; it can only pollute or stain one.

Why is dirt so powerful? And if dirt can be almost anything, how do people recognise it? How do we feel it? The symbol of dirt is recognisable to the body because it affects us. Both the sensory properties of dirt – the ways in which our idea of what dirt is disrupts or interrupts the senses – and our knowledge of what dirt might do or contain – give it emotional and affective power. Outside of the symbolic realm of representational language, the subject recognises dirt in part through how it affects them. And symbols are charged by this meaning intensified in the encounter. As Turner argues, symbols should rally emotion in order to have power, to work (Turner 1967, 29, 36). 'These emotions are portrayed and evoked in close relation to the dominant symbols of tribal cohesion and continuity, often by the performance of instrumentally symbolic behaviour', he argues. 'However, since they are often associated with the mimesis of interpersonal and intergroup conflict, such emotions and acts of behaviour obtain no place among the official, verbal meanings attributed to such dominant symbols' (Turner 1967, 39). The emotional content of symbols is often non-performative, unacknowledged.

This gives these symbols intense emotional power, as they are experienced and felt rather than simply understood or interpreted. For example, the immediate response to a disgust object is automatic, experienced as a compulsion, an imperative. Disgust focuses attention on a perceived threat; it creates an 'intense consciousness' of the object (Tomkins 1962, 128). This physical response can make the meaning ascribed to an object seem 'natural'; something universally bad rather than culturally reviled. The affect of disgust thus makes symbols like dirt and filth matter; it makes them significant to the body, resonant. Yet it is without qualification by language in the first instance. And because this affect is prior to our conscious assessment of the object, because our response to it is embodied before it is qualified, dirt seems disgusting *a priori*. Affect makes the symbol of dirt real to the body rather than an abstract category in the symbolic order.

1.3 Affect Trouble

Debate about the proper use of term 'affect' is currently troubled. A good primer to the debate on 'affect theory' comes from recent discussion of Ruth Ley's critique of the uses (and abuses) of affect theory in the humanities in *The Ascent of Affect* and 'The Turn to Affect: A Critique' (Leys 2011; Leys 2017). Of relevance to this study is Leys' concern with the question of whether affect should be considered autonomic or intentional and her criticism of the 'shared anti-intentionalism' of affect theorists (Leys 2011, 443). She looks to the psychological studies that have been the basis of some of the foundation texts of affect studies, such as Brian Massumi's *The Autonomy of Affect*, to argue that the way he characterises affect as automatic and intense, with an apparent lack of intention, divests it of its historical and cultural agency. Leys is particularly averse to affect theory deriving from Brian Massumi's theory of the autonomy of affect as prior to 'action and expression' and independent of volition and consciousness (Leys 2011, 437; Massumi 2002). She is also critical of Silvan Tomkins, who uses ideas and reports of experiments from evolutionary psychology and neuroscience as a basis of a theory of affect that emerges as a spontaneous and unintentional response to stimuli[2] (Leys 2011, 437–8). What binds these approaches is the claim that 'affect is independent of signification and meaning' (Leys 2017, 314–315). For Leys this is too passive. It denies the ways in which intentions shape our affective responses, creating questions of moral culpability (Leys 2011, 465–8; Leys 2017, 355). I argue – specifically with regard to disgust – that the spontaneity of affect does not occlude intention; it just displaces it in time. I demonstrate this by historicising the terms 'affect' and 'emotion' and by theorising that the disgust reaction can be shaped by what we learn and judge worthy of it in everyday life. In this way we can overcome some of the limits of the use of the term 'affect' in 'affect theory' which derive their authority from potentially flawed experimental models (Leys 2017, 314). Instead, there is an option to restore our sense of the term as one which interrogates the extent to which our responses are influenced by our own intentions and able to be modified by conscious effort when we understand our responses better.

1.4 Historicising Affect

In his 2003 book *From Passions to Emotions: The Creation of a Secular Psychological Category*, historian Thomas Dixon claims the term 'emotion' was an invention of the nineteenth-century secular sciences. With the growth of psychology as a secular science, 'emotion' was adopted as a secular term, and fewer philosophical, metaphysical, or theological psychologies were developed in intellectual contexts (Dixon 2003, 4, 21). In the nineteenth century the taxonomy of feeling terms became more uniform when they were established as universalist categories (Frevert 2016, 52). Frevert argues, '[t]he notion that the body was an unchanging biological entity independent of culture implied that its movements and functions pertained to all human beings' (Frevert 2016, 52). However philosophical reflection on affect and the passions can be traced to uses by Aristotle in ancient Greece, Cicero in classical Rome, the mediaeval scholars Augustine and Aquinas, and were later adapted by enlightenment philosophers Baruch Spinoza and Immanuel Kant, as well as psychoanalytic and postmodern theorists Sigmund Freud and Michel Foucault. Even the question of whether affects are passive or active

---

[2] In this Element I refer to some of Tomkins' descriptions of the disgust reaction without endorsing his contention that disgust is an 'innate affect' (Tomkins 1962).

can be traced all the way back to Aristotle's *De Anima*, in which it was argued that feelings that were closest to God were more active and those that were closest to matter were more passive or involuntary (Dixon 2003, 36). The closest concept to the emotions in Latin or Greek was the concept of the *motus* or *moto dell'anima*, the movement of the soul towards or away from something (Dixon 2003, 39).

In medieval Christian theology, both Augustine and Aquinas seemed to favour a mediated set of affects, one where the spontaneous reactions of the soul were nonetheless subject to reason or rationality with the ultimate aim of virtue (Dixon 2003, 56). Aquinas differentiates the involuntary passions of the soul usually in response to an excitement of the senses from *affectus*, which was more voluntary, stemming from the will or intellect. For Dixon the early signification of this term was not incompatible with intention or influence from the will. In an Aristotelian-Christian framework, affect was a voluntary and impelling force of the will, inherently superior to the involuntary passions of the soul (Dixon 2003, 46). This notion of affect Dixon compares with Augustine's affections, which, unlike passions, were 'voluntary movements of the will, active and ascribable to the angels and to God' (Dixon 2003, 46). In this philosophy, reason and emotions were not averse, and emotion did not necessarily overpower reason. That is, Dixon argues, '[a]ppetites, passions and affections, in the classical Christian view, were all movements of the different parts of the will, and the affections at least were potentially informed by reason' (Dixon 2003, 22).

The use of a wide range of terms to describe physiological, mental, and feeling states, such as passions, emotions, affects, appetites, and drives, produced a diversity of individual, cultural, and historical perspectives, as well as a kind of emotional adaptability. If our conditions could change, then so could the habits mediating our passions, affects, and sensations. Yet the way these different terms mediate between notions of will, reason, and spontaneity – their plasticity – was forgotten or ignored by the psychological sciences, with their focus on reproducibile and universal categories applicable in every historical or cultural context (Frevert 2016, 52). I argue that we should value this nuanced and antique lexicon, which recognises this inherent changeability or 'diachronic and synchronic plasticity', in the dynamic between contemporary research into emotions and the history and anthropology of emotions (Frevert 2016, 53). In the next section I propose a better understanding of the diachronic and synchronic plasticity of disgust.

1.5 Plasticity of Disgust

From their controlled experiments and ethnographic reports, psychologists Paul Rozin and April Fallon conclude that people in every culture likely experience disgust.[3] However, they contend, disgust is always learned. Infants do not express disgust and put vile substances in their mouths. In a controlled study, 62 per cent of infants under the age of two were willing to eat a concoction of peanut butter and smelly cheese modelled as dog faeces, and 31 per cent would eat a whole grasshopper. Only by the age of two do children express distaste, and only by age eight do they express disgust proper (Rozin et al. 1987, 34).

This view is consistent with Kristeva's argument that abjection is a movement that characterises the development of the child. She argues that early emotional responses are only affective, but later become salient, qualified emotional experiences once one becomes a speaking subject who is able to use language or other forms of cultural symbolism. The intervention of language and culture is therefore precisely the way in which we ascribe meaning to these affective states. I maintain in the case of disgust at least there is an indirect relationship between the immediate affective reaction and its emotional qualification. They are interdependent. Carolyn Pedwell has argued by contrast that the turn to affect was not supposed to be at the expense of an understanding of semiotics or signification, but as a compliment to it (Pedwell 2020, 139). Even Boddice and Smith have claimed that while they do not want to maintain a distinction between affect and emotion, they 'remain alive to the non-verbal, and to the body and the brain' (Boddice et al. 2020, 17). The affective, physiological response of disgust should not be considered as independent of meaning, judgement, and intention. In fact, these spontaneous responses are indeed informed by how we think, learn, and evaluate in everyday life.

During a disease outbreak, the category of dirt or what we respond to with aversion will change depending on our certainty or lack of certainty about what constitutes a threat. What belongs to the category of disgust objects is to some extent flexible. In the recent experience of the Covid-19 pandemic, for example, people may have seen others disgusted by the once ordinary task of shaking hands or sitting next to someone on a bus, all the way to the simple act of breathing the same air in a room, particularly with others who were not wearing face masks which inhibit the dispersion of aerosol droplets that might spread a virus. Disgust can apply itself to an almost indefinite range of objects and contexts (Rozin et al. 1987, 34). As it has no absolute identity in and of itself, it must be limited by culture, knowledge, and experience.

---

[3] Jones argues that while disgust appears to be common to all cultures and people, it is impossible to state conclusively that disgust is universal (Jones 2000, 53). However, this view is opposed by epidemiologists such as Valerie Curtis who argue that it is probably disgust is universal to all cultures and histories as an avoidance mechanism for disease vectors in our evolutionary history (Curtis 2007, 661).

Disgust is thus subject to our judgement and discernment. It develops alongside a sense of morality. According to Miller, we learn something, then we learn when to limit or apply the rule. As Douglas would maintain, this ongoing work of culture continuously produces exceptions or borderline cases that defy our efforts at classification (Miller 1997, 14). By way of example, as I explore in Section 4, the New South Wales government decided that all contacts of plague cases had to be quarantined. Plague contacts were treated as abject and literally cast outside the boundaries of the city into a distant quarantine station. That is, until a plague case resulted in quarantine of the entire staff of a hospital, when the rule was lifted in that instance. The hospital staff were too useful to be abject. The presence of these staff was justified because it permitted social life, business, and, in this case, care for people who were likely suffering from diseases more contagious than the bubonic plague (Miller 1997, 14). Likewise, we may learn that a warm temperature indoors indicates a form of cosiness, but that rule may change during a disease outbreak to indicate a lack of fresh air flow and an excess of exhalation, of breathing itself. Our culturally produced faculties of judgement, reason, sense – the symbolic – make often shifting rules or prohibitions which limit and apply our understanding of what is disgusting. As Kristeva says, 'abjection itself is a composite of affect and judgement, of condemnation and yearning, of signs and drives' (Kristeva 1982, 10).

However, several points complicate this issue of evaluation. Emotions and affects can be implicated in and maintained through prereflexive everyday routines which are the product of habit (Bourdieu 1977, 72, 95; Carel 2016, 22). 'To the extent that affect can have an influence automatically – without attention or intention and seemingly irresistibly – it can be understood as a deeply ingrained, overlearned habit, or as a process of chunking and organising a situation' (Isen et al. 1989, 144). These habits make the judgements and evaluations of culture seem commonplace or even inviolable. Yet habits can be challenged if we have new knowledge or information. This can happen frequently in the early stages of a pandemic when knowledge is still in development.

The problem here is not necessarily in drawing a distinction between involuntary, autonomic, affective responses and codified, textual, or symbolic emotions but rather in assuming that they are entirely independent of one another. It is necessary to discover how different affects may or may not be shaped by evocative discourses and instruments of culture, as well as individual learning and experience. In the discourses produced in the first plague outbreak in Sydney, the cultural symbolism of dirt mobilised disgust to advocate for responses suitable to deal with disorder, like sanitation, quarantine, fumigation, and the targeting of specific communities. It also made these arguments affective, so palpable to the body that they seemed to be authorised by nature, independent of the culture and knowledge that was producing them.

1.6 The Ontology of Disgust Objects

So how and why are the things we find disgusting so variable, and so easily applied to other cultures, practices and places? Rozin and Fallon argue almost all cultures find some form of animal product disgusting (Rozin et al. 1987, 28). These items he calls 'primary disgust objects', which disgust without association with other objects. Other items gravitate around this core, becoming disgusting by experience or association. In the Handbook of Emotions, Rozin et al. revised their definition of 'primary disgust objects' to the notion of 'core disgust' (Rozin et al. 2016, 816). Animal or bodily products are usually the basis for disgust – with the exception of tears or milk (Rozin et al. 2016, 818). They maintain the view articulated in their original 1987 study, that there is also a category of metaphoric or symbolic disgust objects or triggers that is derived from this core disgust category and is tremendously variable (Rozin et al. 2016, 829).

The response of disgust appears to be fairly consistent across cultures, perhaps universal. But what occupies the category of disgust object is far more variable, despite efforts to argue that there are primary or core disgust objects based on animal products or the odour of decay (Rozin et al. 2016, 819). There are a wide variety of interpretations and divergences between cultures in what is considered a disgusting sight or odour, as well as their meanings and powers. Indeed, for the symbolic anthropologists Victor Turner and Milton Lewis, olfaction counts as part of the most overlooked but also the most powerful aspect of our symbolic experience. In Alfred Gell's ethnography of the Umeda of Papua New Guinea, odour is identified with giving magic its efficacy or capacity (Gell 1975). Other magic potions such as *Oktesap* infuse the general atmosphere with a specific transformative aroma that is attractive to desirable game and also capable of changing the mental state of the hunter that must pursue it (Lewis 1977, 26). Turner has shown that among the Ndembu of the Congo particularly bad smelling or disgusting herbs are used in medicine in order to drive away illness or disease (Turner 1967, 301). In this instance, the disgusting odour does not provoke distance, but its affective intensity is instrumentalised for its intended healing properties.

There is a dynamic between core and symbolic categories which gives the symbolic its resonance in different settings. But the symbolic or secondary category is culturally variable and not restricted to animal products. Ideas about what constitutes a secondary disgust object and the context to which those objects belong vary considerably across cultures and over time. For Rozin and Fallon, a secondary disgust object is created by 'sympathetic magic', whereby any association, resemblance, or contact between a disgust item and another item has the potential to render the following item disgusting (Rozin et al. 1987, 29–30). The deliberate association of some cultures and identities with dirt and filth resulted in their being regarded as disgust objects. Tomkins refers to the means by which disgust is associated with a variety of objects as the 'similarity principle', because it results from a similarity between a core disgust object and another object, or from contact between them (Tomkins 1962, 130). He argues that we react with disgust to objects that we refuse to smell or eat, due to their similarity to or contact with disgust objects or if we have mixed feelings about an object, such as a mix of fear and desire. We can learn disgust at something which might be similar to a disgust object, he argues, or consciously or unconsciously, when we see disgust expressed, if we identify with the performer (Tomkins 1962, 233). This would be comparable to Mauss' notion that 'techniques of the body' are learned and internalised through mimesis when we observe and value the prestige of the demonstrator (Mauss 1973, 73). An item can be disgusting simply because of the context in which it emerges. According to Rozin and Fallon, chocolate fudge that is shaped as dog faeces disgusts by resemblance; soup stirred by a new fly swatter will disgust by association with its purpose. A tissue left on a table makes both table and tissue disgusting; a tissue in a rubbish bin is more appropriate. Apple juice is not disgusting if it is served in a glass, but if it is served in the wrong context – a urine collection bowl – it can excite disgust (Rozin et al. 1987, 29–30).

The similarity principle can be compared to the qualia of disgust, the more long-term sense of revulsion that people feel in response to one another's conduct or actions (Rozin et al. 2016, 817). This quale both learns from and produces cultural standards, or as Historian Robert J. Kaster claims, the 'symbolic structure' of culture (Kaster 2001, 186). It is therefore particularly important for the work of creating social hierarchy. What Kaster gives us is that what we are disgusted by will depend not only on what we learn to be disgusted by but how we rank, evaluate or scale that person or object. This moral dimension of disgust resonates with the idea of the *scala naturae* from Rozin et al. where in each culture human and non-human beings are ranked in a hierarchy which stretches from pure to impure, sacred to degraded, and those falling towards the base would be conceived as more disgusting (Rozin et al. 2016, 821).

Kaster describes two general forms of disgust reaction also based on the object or stimuli which provoke them. First, the visceral, reflexive, reaction that people have to food, something that would appear to 'arise autonomically', as something independent of will and choice, which he calls the 'per se reflex' (Kaster 2001, 150). This is the one that appears normal or natural and common to all people (Kaster 2001, 185). So 'it unifies you with all the other subjects who are in the same boat when it comes to body – odour, bedbugs or lizards – and to defecation, incest or boasting as well' (Kaster 2001, 186). This is the complete opposite in terms of process from what he argues is the second, more considered response to a wider variety of objects and ethical situations, which he calls the dynamics of 'deliberative ranking', implicated in the establishment of social hierarchies (Kaster 2001, 163).

While there has been no resolute agreement as to the ontology of disgust objects, they are usually described as belonging to two classes, one of which is more symbolic, variable, and cultural. The value of this understanding is that this variability is indexed to the working of the disgust response. The disgust response, in a sense, produces an object as disgusting. Our affective, embodied response will be subject to change according to our mutable definition of what is a disgust object.

1.7 Voluntary Affect

As outlined previously, the cultural processes and ideas that inform the disgust response do not have a start and end point; they are more circular than linear. While disgust identifies an object as disgusting, it also makes that object noticeable. The affect of disgust is daily informed by conscious and unconscious evaluations that are elemental to every culture. It is mediated by culture. Yet there is a time lapse between affect and judgement, affect is immediate, judgement mostly occurs more slowly, during everyday life. In Section 3, I will explain in more detail how cultural judgement operates regarding the category of secondary or symbolic disgust objects. By focusing on our responses to symbols and by arguing that our everyday evaluations and judgements influence our affective responses, I hope to overcome this strict demarcation of affect as completely involuntary and irresponsible, showing indeed that specific affects like disgust are rather more complicated in how they interact with judgement and the symbolic.

Bettina Hitzer's research on the recent history of cancer treatment in German hospitals shows us the changing threshold of tolerance to the smell of the cancerous body and the use of odour as an indicator to diagnose the severity of cancer (Hitzer 2020, 163). Hitzer argues that there is some medical literature which identifies the disgust felt by medical professionals and trains them to mask it (Hitzer 2020, 158). For Sarah-Maria Schober the capacity to overcome disgust has historically been instrumentalised by medical practitioners to demonstrate their experience with the medical arts of surgery and dissection (Schober 2020, 49).

She claims early modern medical anatomists like Felix Platter deliberately engaged in disgusting practices such as consumption of bodily products to establish an 'anatomical persona' which qualified them for the practice of medicine (Schober 2020, 48–49). However, she does not necessarily maintain that practitioners who advocated disgusting treatment such as the consumption of bodily discharge were not aware of what they were doing or did not themselves – at least initially – find these treatments disgusting. While these practitioners may have been able to recognise objects as disgusting, they were able to overcome this recognition, which is to say to transform the affective response of disgust in order to demonstrate their capability (Schober 2020, 49). These arguments illustrate my point that it is possible to consciously inform ourselves how to respond to some things and to overcome – at least to some extent – our spontaneous reactions of disgust. This is because disgust is a learned response, as Rozin and Fallon claim, one subject to cultural evaluation.

Disgust can be instrumentalised, made direct use of, in order to attract the attention and interest of readers (Schober 2020, 49). Schober describes anatomists like Christian Franz Paullini, author of *Heylsame Dreckapotheke* or *Curative Dirt Apothecary*, who described eating dirt as a form of treatment, even though he knew it would repulse his readers, which was a deliberate strategy to attract interest and demonstrate the productivity of disgust (Schober 2020, 51–2). She refers to this duality as the 'paradox of disgust', a common rhetorical strategy in early modern medicine, as 'disgust remained at this time sufficiently ambivalent an emotion that scientists and successful merchants could use it effectively to promote their activities, products and even themselves' (Schober 2020, 50).

If how we relate to objects and identities is learnt, then it can be re-learnt with intention. What people respond to with disgust is not fixed but is subject to change according to the specificity of culture, history, and individual personality. By engaging with discourse, by communicating with one another, by watching and learning, we see what others find disgusting and learn to be disgusted by it too. In Sydney in 1900, both official and vernacular discourse used dirt endlessly to fill in the gaps in uncertain medical knowledge and to channel and provoke affect. Particularly regarding the fumigation of the city and sanitation, we can see the plasticity of the disgust response at work in Sydney in 1900.

1.8 Sources and Evidence

The third global plague pandemic was remarkable for the way in which data regarding epidemiology, transmission and containment was produced and shared (Anon, 1907, 60; Ashmead 1901, 9). It coincided with the early development of international public health architecture designed to systematise the reporting and monitoring of the disease's spread. An international sanitary conference in 1897 focused exclusively on plague for the first time. This Venice Plague Conference produced an international convention that provided for worldwide notification of new plague outbreaks. Thus from 1894 the New South Wales Board of Health began to issue special resolutions and directions in response to the plague pandemic as it spread to India and other ports such as Mauritius, Reunion, and Seychelles (Ashburton-Thompson 1900b, 13–14). Even before the pandemic reached Sydney, the notification system led to the production and communication of data. The publication and distribution of epidemiological reports in international journals sustained the Australian press and other discursive producers like politicians with ongoing stories of the outbreaks in different ports, cities, and colonies.

This data is a useful source for analysis. I use public health reports from Australia and England, records of parliamentary debates and speeches, complaints to council, letters to the editor, newspaper articles, advertisements and reports of the cleaning operations conducted by the government appointed architect George McCredie, including the collection of photographs he made to justify his interventions across the city. Many of these photos were taken at the time as a form of collateral. The cleaning and sanitation crews often destroyed properties and there were complaints about their activities, as documented in Section 4 (see Figure 1). Some of McCredie's photos are reproduced in this Element, to show how different agents attempted to frame the city as incorrigibly dirty and in need of change. I analyse the authorisation of power using affective symbols in these texts, and indicators of non-compliance. My sources are mostly of literate Anglophone men in public life who produced discourse to solicit affect and convey their emotions. The voices of people who did not have means or capability to publish their views in English are fewer, except where they have participated in institutions or been quoted by journalists and politicians. Indigenous voices and the voices of the Chinese and immigrants from outside the British Empire are regrettably absent. While the sources are limited, I do identify some discord or heterogeneity about the optimal course of action and resistance to the public health measures within these texts.

As William Reddy has argued, a historical anthropology of the emotions requires working with textual sources, which – rightly or wrongly – may imply more certainty and less confusion, incoherence and obfuscation than an observation of speech and gesture (Reddy 1997, 346). Yet even within these texts there is evidence of heterogeneity and disagreement. As Boddice and Hitzer argue, it is important not to take historical sources at face value but to

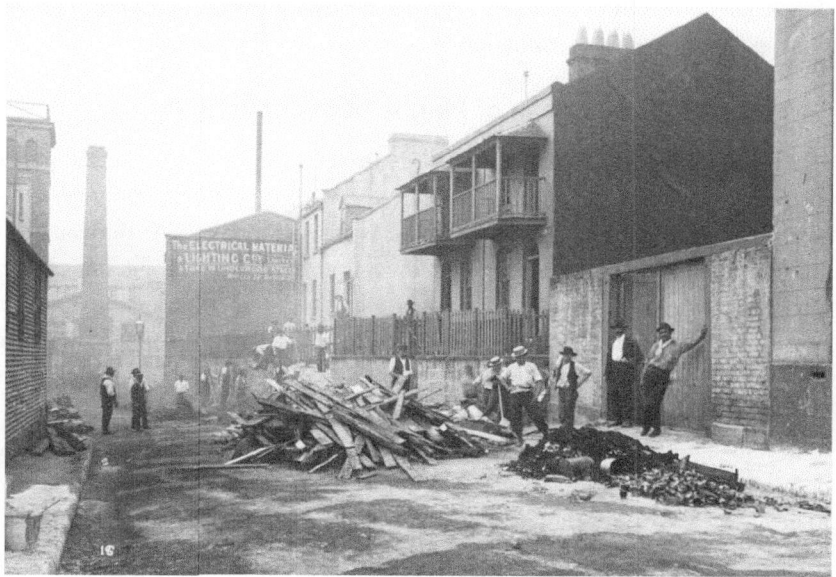

Figure 1 Views taken during cleansing operations, Napoleon Street, Sydney, 1900, Vol. I. Under the supervision of Mr George McCredie, NSW. 1900. Image courtesy: Collections of the State Library of New South Wales.

understand their overt and covert complexity and multiplicity (Boddice et al. 2022, 10). These differences of opinion were audible even in the dominant discourses in conflicts between the Chief Health Officer of NSW Ashburton-Thompson and the NSW Premier William Lyne over whether the disease was contagious and people in contact with the sick should be quarantined; the initial reluctance of people to work on the cleaning crews, followed by the clamour to do so; the vitriolic racism against the Chinese; the satirising of the fear and apprehension of the public to things like touching money, walking past people on the sidewalk, or kissing the Bible in court; and the arguments between the state government and municipal council over who was responsible for reform.

To resolve uncertainties, fill in gaps in logic, or advocate for a specific course of action, these accounts frequently resorted to the symbolism of dirt, which provoked disgust and other affects. As Victor Turner claims, 'the significant elements of a symbol's meaning are related to what it does and what is done to it by and for whom' (Turner 1967, 46). Some symbols are received and interpreted without having been intended; yet they still condition experience. They are subject to cultural and historical change, and their use is an exercise of power. The duality of dirt and the abject was simultaneously repulsive and fascinating to draw the interest of readers in 1900, and to authorise the response

they believed was most adequate, whether it was repression of specific populations, particular kinds of sanitation or other coercive measures.

2 Outbreak of Plague at Sydney, 1900

At the end of the nineteenth century, lorry driver Arthur Payne collected goods
from the docks at Darling Harbour in the growing port city of Sydney, the
capital of the British colony of New South Wales, in Australia. As thirteen ships
arrived from overseas 'plague ports' like Bombay, Hong Kong, Singapore,
Honolulu, and Nouméa, where the disease had been reported, infected rats on
board one or several of these vessels jumped ship. By early 1900 plague had
begun to spread among the local city rats and their fleas in Sydney. Payne was
the first to be infected.

In mid-January, he was suddenly seized with giddiness and headache as he
delivered cargo to a warehouse in the city. Once he arrived back at work, he had
to lie down. After a few hours, he felt a strange aching lump in his left thigh. At
home later his symptoms worsened; he became feverish, and occasionally
vomited. His temperature reached 40.5 Celsius, his pulse raced. By the following morning, Payne's face was flushed and puffy, and he gazed out at the world
from watery, suffused eyes. A gland in his left upper thigh swelled to the size of
an almond, becoming tender and painful. Two days later doctors found near his
Achilles' tendon a purplish red wound about 3 mm in diameter, where he may
have been bitten by a flea. They suspected plague. On the 19th of January 1900,
the 33-year-old was the first in Sydney to be diagnosed with the bubonic plague.
Fortunately, over the next few days, their patient seemed to recover. He was pale
and tremulous for a while, but his temperature slowly went down and he was
finally able to get some sleep (Ashburton-Thompson 1900b, 77–8). The city
relaxed with him. As Arthur Payne recovered, the public barely registered
a threat. While Sydney's 1900 plague outbreak might have begun with Arthur
Payne, according to William Hughes, the first case of plague 'passed almost
without notice' in the eyes of the public. Until mid-February, when Captain
James Ridley Dudley died (New South Wales Parliament 1900a, 208).

It may be unfair to impute ulterior motives to Mrs Dudley or to doubt her
clinical judgement. Yet the wife of the second case, or 'alleged case' of plague,
Captain Dudley, wrote to the authorities with 'some excellent reasons', according to parliamentarian William Hughes, why her husband could not have had
a 'genuine case' of the plague. She believed, and Hughes did not contradict her,
that it was instead misdiagnosed peritonitis (New South Wales Parliament
1900a, 208). Captain Dudley was a sailmaker who worked on local vessels
coming and going from Darling Harbour. Three days before he became ill,

Dudley fell, hitting a plank and injuring his abdomen. He was visited by three doctors and diagnosed with septic fever. The Chief Medical Officer and President of the New South Wales Board of Health, Dr Ashburton-Thompson stated confidently that no peritonitis was suspected. On February 23rd Dudley died. Noticing his swollen inguinal glands, the doctors suspected plague. They removed them for laboratory tests. As soon as an hour later, they quarantined the staff and residents on the second storey of the building at 47–57 Sussex Street, where he ran his business. They also spoke to several of his staff. These incarcerated 'inmates' reported that Dudley had himself removed five dead rats from a water closet 'connected in a primitive fashion' with a pipe drain discharging sewerage to the harbour a few days before he died (Ashburton-Thompson 1900b, 79).

For Ashburton-Thompson, Dudley's drain was a kind of concierge inviting diseased rats disembarking from foreign ships to do business in Sydney. But his opinion was not conclusive evidence. That would come from Sydney's first government bacteriologist, Dr Frank Tidswell. When he received a new specimen and clinical evidence of potential plague, either from a human or rat, Dr Tidswell initially examined it under a microscope. If the results supported plague, he proceeded to conduct two further tests, called cultural and inoculation tests. Positive results allowed for a definite diagnosis of plague. By the day after Dudley died, Tidswell reported that he had obtained positive results from all three tests of Dudley's femoral and inguinal buboes (Ashburton-Thompson 1900b, 50).

Mrs Dudley's defences may have been prompted by shame at the enormous crowd of police which surrounded her home in Drummoyne after her husband's death. As William Reddy argues, shame derives from our perception of how we are seen by others. 'Thus, shame can lead to withdrawal coupled with action aimed at managing appearances' (Reddy 1997, 347). But appearances were hard to manage in this case, Mr Reid claimed, 'one could not even get to the fence' of her house, while a little boathouse nearby was also surrounded by policemen. As another parliamentarian interjected, his 'yacht was quarantined also' (New South Wales Parliament 1900a, 208). At home in Drummoyne, Mrs Dudley readily publicised that she had done her best to reduce risk and keep a clean household, perhaps to avoid being labelled irresponsible. Three weeks before her husband fell ill and died, Hughes reported, she is said to have written to the municipal council to ask for a 'heap of rubbish' to be removed from a blind alley near her house. William Hughes clarified, 'I do not mean a heap as big as a cathedral, but I mean a heap so big that those of us who are here might easily have been buried underneath it . . . composed of rotten bananas, bagging, and the various kind of flotsam and jetsam that accumulate about the wharves of

Sydney.' For Hughes, the odours reeking from this heap of composting refuse were 'a congenial nest, a hotbed, a ferment' for the 'germs of plague flying around' (New South Wales Parliament 1900a, 209). In reports that were challenged in parliament as 'exaggerated', tons of rubbish were removed from the laneway weeks after Dudley's death by the government's specially appointed plague quarantine and cleaning crew, headed by architect George McCreadie (New South Wales Parliament. 1860, 209). By March the City of Sydney had been directed by the secretary of the Board of Health to serve a notice on the landlord, one honourable Jon See, to reconstruct the sewerage connection (Secretary, Dept. of Public Health 1900).

Irrespective of Mrs Dudley's obvious shame, and her attempts to displace responsibility for the presence of rats onto the local council, some parliamentarians implicated the condition of Dudley's workplace in his eventual susceptibility to disease. They lambasted the government and Board of Health for sending so many police officers to his household while quarantining only one level of his workplace. The basement of his building in Sussex Street had 'all the conditions for rats and the harbouring of disease', claimed parliamentarian Mr Reid (New South Wales Parliament 1900a, 80). The second storey of the building where Mr Dudley had his sailmaker business 'was a damp, dark, badly ventilated place, with drainage oozing through one of the walls'. Underneath Dudley on the first floor was the office of shipping company John See & Co and a produce store, and beneath all of them a 'dark, damp, badly ventilated cellar'. In April, over a month after Dudley died, Reid alleged, the cellar still harboured a 'large quantity of rotting mouldy straw, and there was an accumulation of cobwebs and dirt of every kind'. Mr Reid quoted from a report supposedly created by the cleaning crew, which reported that they had '[r]emoved large quantities of filth from area window, the glass of which was completely obscured by dirt'. However, he was discredited in the assembly for not tabling the report or revealing the name of the author (New South Wales Parliament 1900a, 81). The impetuous Reid insisted that the Board of Health should have evicted every business from the building and had 'everything taken out and burnt' (New South Wales Parliament 1900a, 83).

The entire district around Sussex Street where Dudley worked and lived some of the time was quarantined following his death, while the plague 'proceeded zigzag across Sussex-street to three or four places' before jumping streets to spread further into the city and along the harbourside wharves (New South Wales Parliament 1900a, 208). Nearby residents scrambled to disassociate themselves. The *Sydney Morning Herald* reported that a Mr Durrell lived only 50 yards or so from Dudley, but after Mr Durrell objected, the paper revised its statement to say that he lived a full 200 yards away (Sydney

Morning Herald 1900a, 3). Being quarantined for intervention was embarrassing, inconvenient and could result in property and entire homes being destroyed by cleaning crews. Individuals, families, houses, shops, and suburbs all made valiant efforts to avoid plague itself and its shameful associations (see Figure 2).

When a limited supply of 'Haffkine's prophylactic' was made available for vaccination on March 21st, the public reacted with anxiety and panic. In a speech to parliament in June, William Hughes recalls the reaction of the public to Dudley's death and the subsequent limited provision of vaccines,

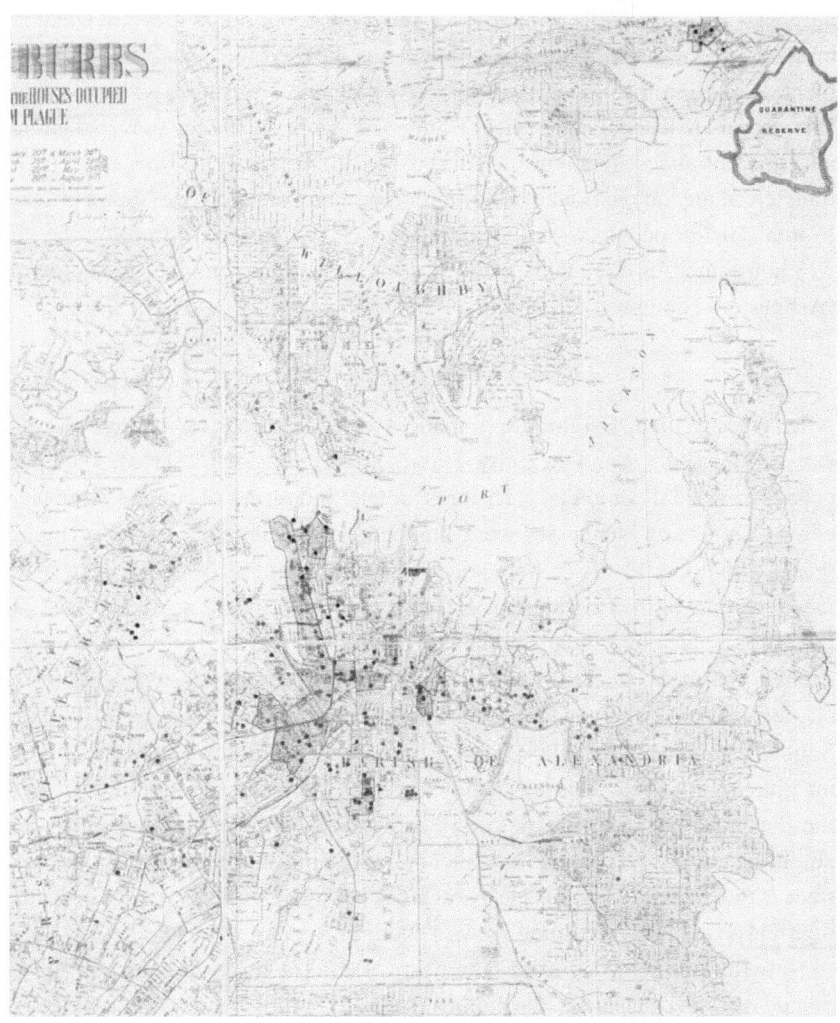

Figure 2 Map of Sydney and suburbs showing by coloured spots the positions of the houses occupied by 294 persons who suffered from plague. Image courtesy: Collections of the State Library of New South Wales.

the Board of Health building had almost been demolished piecemeal, and when I went there next day, it was a ruin. Thousands of people had attempted to get in by main force, men and women had fainted, people had climbed in through the windows; the whole place was simply on the eve of a great panic, in fact in my opinion, the panic had set in. (New South Wales Parliament 1900a, 209)

At this point the Premier William Lyne interjected, to point out that the public broke the staircase of the Board of Health building. In Ashburton-Thompson's account, 'the public, without any warning, suddenly arrived in very great numbers and practically took possession of the building; they invaded the upper part of it, packing the staircases almost beyond the possibility of movement, and at imminent risk of a disastrous accident', while those waiting outside 'desperately resisted displacement from positions of advantage they had gained near the entrances' (Ashburton-Thompson 1900b, 19). The Board of Health transferred the inoculation to an exhibition building at the Sydney Showground. In total 10,700 people were inoculated, which Ashburton-Thompson claimed was not numerous enough to interfere with the natural course of the epidemic (Ashburton-Thompson 1900b, 11).

2.1 'City of the Dead'

After Dudley died, Sydneysiders made a considerable effort to put distance between themselves and their city. Sydney was completely deserted. The upper classes avoided it completely. Theatres, hotels, and places of congregation were empty. Shops and businesses were shunned. As parliamentarian Billy Hughes recalled in June, in the initial stages of the pandemic, '[p]eople were being frightened out of their seven senses' (New South Wales Parliament 1900a, 210). For Hughes even by June the population of Sydney had not recovered from this catalytic moment, 'there are many people, who are generally residents of the city and suburbs, who have not yet mustered up the courage to come back' (New South Wales Parliament 1900a, 209). An advertisement for The Mutual Stores on Pitt Street stated, 'Owing to the scare caused by the Plague, numbers of families have been kept away from the city, and visitors from the country and adjoining colonies have been conspicuous in their absence. The consequence to trade is that there is a surplusage in our stocks of winter articles, especially of the high-class qualities' (Evening News 1900d, 8).

Notwithstanding Ashburton-Thompson's efforts to assure the public the plague was not contagious, the public responded to the plague with considerable fear and aversion, which compelled them to distance themselves from the location of the supposed threat. In Sydney, the constant threat of disease made the population diffident in its dealings with each other, while the plague epidemic generated outright hostility. People could not confidently interact with each other, without fearing that someone or other might harbour the inconspicuous germs that would cause them harm. Rather than venture to the city, people found new ways to do business, placing orders through postcards, letters, telegrams, and telephone. In March, the *Evening News* visited the wholesale district of the city to gauge the 'public feeling' regarding the progress of the plague, reporting 'when a Sussex Street merchant meets a customer in other parts of the city, discusses business, and winds up with a trite saying: "Will you call at my office?" a frequent rejoinder is: "I would rather telephone"' (Evening News 1900b, 6). Distance was an imperative.

The seventh Australian Prime Minister William M. Hughes, who was a member of the New South Wales Parliament in 1900, claimed in a speech to the Legislative Assembly, 'if one is to understand what a "city of the dead" would actually be like, I can only state that it would be like the busiest thoroughfare in Sydney, as I knew it for six weeks'. He went on, 'we must remember that there was a panic – that every man, or nearly every man that could afford it, left Sydney – that thousands of visitors who were coming here avoided Sydney as if it were leprous' (New South Wales Parliament 1900a, 208). Some people went as far as the Blue Mountains, to the west of Sydney. *The Bulletin* stated, 'there is much panic, a mad rush to the Blue Mountains', while the *Sydney Morning Herald* commented 'The truism that "it is an ill wind that blows nobody good" has been exemplified in a marked degree by the benefit accorded the western suburbs through the exodus of the population westward from the city' (The Bulletin 1900b, 6; Sydney Morning Herald 1900e, 10).

While contact with almost anybody was to be avoided, contact with categories of people like the urban poor, recently recovered, or non-British immigrants was repugnant. Some of these people were hauled before the courts for their allegedly degenerate behaviour. A boy of eleven was charged with scattering rubbish in the Water Police Court, after raking through a rubbish box from a shopkeeper on Elizabeth Street. Apparently the boy worked in a team with two or three other smaller children, who, using a handcart, 'raked about in all the rubbish boxes they passed, and when near Hunter Street upset two boxes on the footway, scattering jam tins, banana skins, bottles and rubbish generally all about the place' (Australian Star 1900b, 5). When the Bankruptcy Court was informed that a witness had recently been released from quarantine, the Bible he had kissed was disposed of and another one fetched for the next witness (Evening News 1900c, 6).

For those who were forced to stay in the city, the association of their suburb with a case of plague could cause shame and inconvenience (see Figure 3). The disgrace of association with plague had concrete ramifications, such as quarantine,

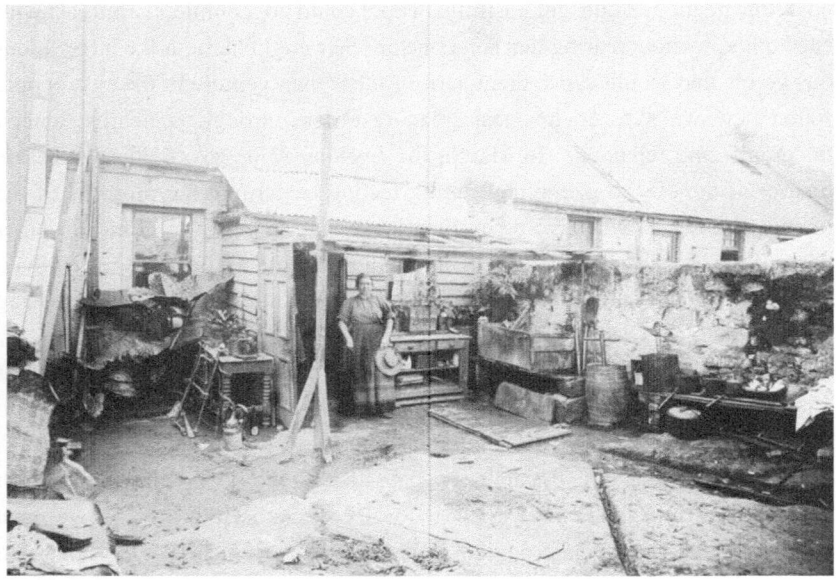

Figure 3 Woman at rear of house, 1 Church Street, Pyrmont [A-00036123]. City of Sydney Demolition Books, 1900. Image courtesy: City of Sydney Archives.

aggressive cleaning, or demolition. One woman from the poorer classes living in the city claimed in a letter that her 'only safety is in cleanliness', a safety she produced with an hour a day of ritual scrubbing of the floors. 'I wish all our neighbours were as clean as we are,' she said. 'We should not fear the plague then. I think the inspectors should go round, accompanied by lady inspectors, and see that all the dwelling rooms are clean' (Evening News 1900b, 6). The fear of contamination and the shame of association were so intense that people evaded the houses and streets of plague cases (whose names and addresses were published in newspapers), informed on people they suspected were ill, and agitated for the removal of those in contact with the sick to quarantine (Curson et al. 1989, 158). Entire suburbs could be corrupted. One newspaper correspondent defined all of Redfern, Annandale, Drummoyne, and the Children's Hospital in Glebe as 'tainted' with the plague (Sydney Morning Herald 1900d, 8). On the 20th of April the *Sydney Morning Herald* published an amendment and apology, claiming that a recent case had been wrongly attributed to the borough of Alexandria, when it actually belonged to an adjacent area (Sydney Morning Herald 1900f, 3). Individuals scurried to disassociate themselves and their localities from the plague and to transform their locality into one which would be considered 'clean'.

While various sites of the city were associated with dirt or disease, trains, trams, and buses were thresholds and intermediaries between the sites. Their indeterminate status led to a variety of complaints as passengers from across the city mixed in unpalatable ways. Newspapers and the Railway Commissioners received complaints about how sick people should not be allowed to travel. A person apparently suffering disease was placed in the second-class carriage of the southern train at Redfern, complained one letter to the editor of *The Cumberland Argus*, while another man boarded a train at Granville station with an asylum attendant. The author objected, '[t]he sufferer's cough was pitiable, and his expectorations disgusting – but the passengers had to put up with both' (Cumberland Argus 1900, 3).

This is not to say that everyone in Sydney adopted the same point of view on the level of risk, or that responses were homogenous. Local satirical magazine *The Bulletin*, at the time the highest selling national publication, published editorials and commentary throughout the plague mocking government and public health practices and extremes of the public reaction. '[T]his is a great time for drunks', it declared in April. 'Any drunk who says that he has a pain in the groin can have the Sydney pavement all to himself to recover on' (The Bulletin 1900c, 10).

The actual number of infections and mortalities from plague was low compared to other diseases in nineteenth-century Sydney, such as diarrhoea, bronchitis, gastroenteritis, venereal disease, dysentery, and tuberculosis (Curson 1985, 91). Yet as the historians Alison Bashford and Carolyn Strange have argued, 'explaining public health policy of the past purely in medical or epidemiological terms ignores evidence that it was rarely, if ever, designed solely on medical grounds at the time' (Bashford et al. 2007, 87). Bettina Hitzer agrees the level of threat accorded to a disease or its emotional impact does not always correspond practically to the number of people who fall ill or die (Hitzer 2022, 63). As medical geographer Peter Curson argues, the public perception of and reaction to the disease is just as important as its impact in how it is framed, 'a handful of plague or smallpox cases in a large city may be regarded as an epidemic simply because of the emotional reaction engendered by the disease' (Curson 1985, 2). It was because of the proliferation of symbolism and emotion, rather than real threat, that the 1900 plague provoked by far the most extreme institutional response among the public of any nineteenth-century epidemic.

3 The Symbolism of Dirt in Discursive Responses to Plague

Many of these discourses attempted to make themselves more authoritative by enlisting the affect of disgust and the symbolism of dirt to compel a physical response in their reader and to intervene in the plasticity of the disgust response – either by downplaying the risk, as we see in the article from *The*

Bulletin, or by heightening our sensitivity to dirt and the risk of disease, to promote a course of action or inaction.

Even Ashburton-Thompson himself was not above such tactics to persuade authorities of the need to demolish the slums.

> It may not look as bad as a London slum, perhaps; but this is merely because of our more liberal sunlight and clearer atmosphere. This collection of filthy black huts – I cannot call them houses, and all other such places are as discovered, will be presented by the medical officer of health for the metropolitan district to the local authority as places unfit for human habitation. They are simply ghastly. (The Bulletin 1900b, 7)

His perturbation was minor compared to the horror and disgust of a plucky journalist, who rolled up his sleeves, held his breath and dived into the WC of one house in the Rocks. In his account, the basin was cracked, the taps were out of order, and the WC was blocked, causing the pan to fill with 'foetid brown excrement'. Worse, when someone attempted to relieve the blockage 'the amount of stinking PUTRIFYING, PESTIFEROUS BLACK OOZE and filth that the writer, handkerchief over nose, saw scooped out of that trap was a caution to snakes … and caused violent vomiting to those engaged in it' (The Truth 1900b, 7). Like Ashburton-Thompson, the author concluded by demanding the demolition of all 'rampantly repulsive' premises.

It was Chinese immigrants that were most heavily targeted by social and institutional practices of aversion and control in response to the plague. In the very centre of the central business district of Sydney, nearby the harbour, up to 1,500 Chinese people lived in 394 houses, working as merchants, cabinet makers, or carpenters, selling fruit or operating restaurants (Curson et al. 1989, 96). The 1891 census recorded nearly 36,000 Chinese immigrants in Sydney, though by 1902 numbers had declined to less than 30,000. Population decline was a result of repressive immigration legislation such as the 1881 Influx of Chinese Restriction Act (New South Wales), which permitted only one person from China to disembark for every hundred tonnes of cargo, on condition they pay a ten-pound poll tax (Manderson 1997, 387). This later became the basis of the country's infamous 'White Australia' policy, the Immigration Restriction Act legislated by the new Commonwealth government in 1901.

The Anglophone press accused various non-English cultures of immorality and degeneracy (Manderson 1997, 386). The *Australian Star* warned that a new case in Redfern indicated it was a seat of infection, made more serious due to its proximity to the 'area occupied by a large number of Asiatics' (Australian Star 1900a, 5). At a meeting in April a City of Sydney Alderman raged, 'The Chinese do not bury their dead-they pickle them and send them home to their ancestors'

(Daily Telegraph 1900, 7). Sydney newspaper *The Truth* was explicit in its association of Chinese bodies with plague threat through the mobilisation of disgust:

> The vegetable den of a Chinaman, the pickle factory of a Syrian, the fruit shop of an Italian, the fish shop of a Greek, the crimping den of a German housekeeper on the waterfront – these are the weak points in Sydney's sanitary system. But with proper municipal and Government regulation, these frowsy foreigners would not be allowed to convert parts of the city into plague spots, to keep cellars full of the offal of fish and poultry, or of decaying vegetables and fruit; or to wallow in personal customs of unmentionable filthiness. (The Truth 1900a, 1)

The archives of the City of Sydney municipal council contain hundreds of complaints requesting the intervention of council during the plague. On 26th of July, John Garland and John J. Cohen wrote a complaint to the City of Sydney complaining of orange skins, vegetable matter, and even human excreta dumped on the Hay Street pathway after the Belmore Markets near Darling Harbour on Saturdays. The cause, it admonished, was that Chinese people were not allowed to use the public toilets, recommending that the council especially erect or set aside some conveniences. 'It is almost impossible to treat these complaints seriously,' retorted the council's City Cleansing Department, arguing that sweeping out the market was 'Monday's work' and that it was not necessary to remove rubbish on a Sunday while it was 'fresh and inoffensive'. On the topic of the toilets, they responded that both the Chinese and Europeans used the existing accommodations, because '[a]ny person who understands the habits of the Chinese knows well that to erect a convenience exclusively for their use would be to offer the very best opportunity for an exhibition of the very filthiest habits it is possible to conceive' (Town Clerk's Correspondence Folders 26th July 1900c).

The extreme associations of Chinese immigrants with dirt, filth, or even faeces during the plague were a form of strategic mobilisation of disgust to justify purgative interventions such as demolition, aversion, disassociation or even inaction. On the 23rd of April the *Sydney Morning Herald* reported that a Chinese man who was sick with the plague had been wrongly attributed to Botany, in spite of the fact that 'so far there has not been a single case within the boundaries of the municipality' (Sydney Morning Herald 1900g, 8). In response, the council arranged for the mayor to inspect each house occupied by Chinese people. His inspection report apparently found their homes to be internally clean and featuring nothing that might be detrimental to the heath of their occupants 'in consequence of their natural habits'. However, the report concluded that each of their homes lacked proper drainage and might therefore 'menace the health of people living in surrounding districts'. To allay panic, Botany Council resolved to condemn the buildings. The demolition of houses in Botany inhabited by the Chinese was an attempt to disassociate the suburb from being defined as the source of contagion, deserving of further interventionist measures of the state. The Chinese and their supposedly irredeemable premises were scapegoated as the source of contagion so their neighbours could live without intervention.

The common racism published by the tabloids was reproduced in a less hysterical form in medical and administrative discourses that struggled to identify an empirical basis for these taken-for-granted hierarchies. Ashburton-Thompson separated Chinese people in his epidemiological data, believing that their customs, diet, and race made them and the other British colonies like India more susceptible to disease. Of the ten Chinese people who were afflicted with the plague, eight died. This mortality rate of 80 per cent was for Ashburton-Thompson proof of the strength of 'whites' which suffered a mortality rate of 34 per cent (Ashburton-Thompson 1900b, 9). In his view this was due to 'the indirect influence of local conditions of life – of feeding, housing, cleanliness, and also of race' (Ashburton-Thompson 1900b, 7). Citing this apparent susceptibility, the Board of Health gave itself a mandate to take a more coercive approach with Chinese populations. For example, it removed Chinese contacts more frequently to quarantine, where they were forcibly vaccinated and segregated in tents nearby the people from European backgrounds, who stayed in buildings. In the city, the homes of the Chinese were also far more likely to be condemned for demolition. In the western Sydney suburb of Parramatta, a meeting of the council heard a report tabled by the Inspector of Nuisances that found most properties in good sanitary condition, except for those of 'a number of Chinamen' in Philip Street, which should be pulled down in the interests of public safety. The council adopted the report and decided to demolish the properties (Evening News 1900a, 6).

The racism felt by Chinese immigrant communities during the plague was not confined to Sydney. Reinarz has documented racism against immigrant Chinese communities across Europe and North America in the nineteenth century, such as in Vancouver, where immigrant communities were described as 'foul-smelling, disease-threatening and dirty' (Reinarz 2014, 100). In his examination of the San Francisco Pesthouse, Guenter Risse identifies how newspaper reports elicited strong emotional responses such as fear, disgust, and anxiety to the physical symptoms of various diseases – in particular focusing on the role of skin conditions and skin diseases in linking the diseased and racialised body. Risse documents 'the plasticity and contingency of emotion-driven behaviours as they manifest themselves in the moral and political judgments that human beings make in confronting and seeking to control contagious diseases' (Risse 2015, 3).This concurs with Hitzer's focus on how disgust was deployed in hygienic campaigns and rhetoric in order to mobilise attention with regard to understandings of cancer in nineteenth-century Germany. She thinks that there was evidence that exhibitions 'instrumentalised visual disgust but also disgusting smells and fears of contamination, and this despite the by then well-known fact that cancer is not contagious' (Hitzer 2020, 161).

Historian Robert Jütte also identifies disgusting odours with the denigration of race and as a justification for racial prejudice in countries like pre-WWII Germany, South Africa during apartheid, and the United States pre- and post-abolition, to justify policies of spatial segregation (Jütte 2018, 174). Classen et al. identify how the odours characterised as belonging to groups defined as racially other can be portrayed as both distinctive and disagreeable, justifying avoidance behaviour (Classen et al. 1994, 165). Bettina Hitzer applies the term 'scandalised illness' from medical historian Alfons Labisch to describe the difference between perception and actual threat, or the way the effects of disease can be projected onto vulnerable groups who are made responsible for them (Hitzer 2022, 63). As psychologist Silvan Tomkins has established, as disgust is usually limited and applied in accordance with cultural understandings, any prejudice can be transformed into disgust as we can learn to interpret any difference between individuals as disgusting (Tomkins 1962, 135). The reaction may be particularly extreme regarding an odour, which need only be intense or strange for us to learn to be disgusted by it. For Tomkins, we can learn to be disgusted with 'any strong odour as such, all the way to any semblance of randomness, noise or disorder in the world' (Tomkins 1962, 235).

Both Smith and Reinarz have argued that from the late nineteenth century odour was increasingly called on as a biological marker of racial difference, as it was supposed to provide data on identity, character and morality, as well as health and ethnic origin (Reinarz 2014, 160; Smith 2018b, 188). Yet it is not the actual smell which 'triggers the experience of difference', as Classens and Howes argue, but that the odour of the other is a feeling of prejudice 'transposed into the 'olfactory domain' as 'smell provides a potent symbolic means for creating and enforcing class and ethnic boundaries' (Classen et al. 1994, 169). This argument would appear to align with the conclusions from the empirical research of historian Bettina Hitzer, who notes that the smells that trigger disgust will change over time (Hitzer 2020, 164). She prefers a historically and culturally specific approach to defining both disgust objects and their sensory qualities, while distinguishing the moral understandings that inform disgust as altogether separate if mutually influential (Hitzer 2020, 158).

The fear provoked by the plague outbreak prompted an intense reaction in public, medical and media discourses, which used the symbolism of dirt and filth to evoke disgust and justify targeted racist interventions against local Chinese populations. In Australia, as Anderson argues, colonial medicine was a form of 'material power that operates on distinctly racial bodies to produce the sort of body that colonial society required' (Anderson 1995, 645). This resulted in a dependence on coercive practices of quarantine and disinfection which targeted non-British races (Anderson 1995, 645). As many new immigrants to Sydney may have discovered in 1900, shared disgust at their customs and even diet may have contributed to the cohesion of an otherwise fragmented settler-colonial class.

4 Development of a City

Prior to the Federation of Australia as a Commonwealth on the 1st of January 1901, Australia was divided into six British colonies. In Sydney, government authority was distributed between the government of the colony of New South Wales and the municipal councils. With the establishment of a central police force in 1862, the New South Wales Government formalised a monopoly of legitimate violence (Hirst 1988, 218–20). Their calculable control over legitimate force pacified the public spaces of the city. This made interactions more predictable because of the belief that the state would intervene to stop any violent or threatening individual.

There were still a number of hazards to contend with in the urban environment. By 1900, the newer houses in the suburbs were mostly all connected to the sewerage network that had been constructed in 1891 (see Figure 4). Ashburton-Thompson noted in one of his own reports that the problems with sewerage in the city of Sydney were not evident in the metropolitan or suburban districts, where 38,000 houses containing 182,000 persons were connected to a sewerage network properly maintained by the Metropolitan Board of Water Supply and Sewerage (Ashburton-Thompson 1900a, 20). Yet back in the city, shared cesspits and water closets were a constant part of everyday life. In many places water closets were directly connected to the mains water, polluting drinking supplies with human waste. The sewers themselves purged contaminated wastewater into Sydney Harbour at multiple points, many of which were located around the city (Fitzgerald 1987, 83). Fetid, stinking waste flowed into gutters on the streets and through a labyrinthine network of open drains and sewers, weaving in and out of city streets to the sea. On the ebb and flow of the harbour tides, the rubbish spread tens of kilometres up the coastline. People living in the city and residents of the suburbs visiting the theatre, going to work, or shopping at department stores had to put up with shit.

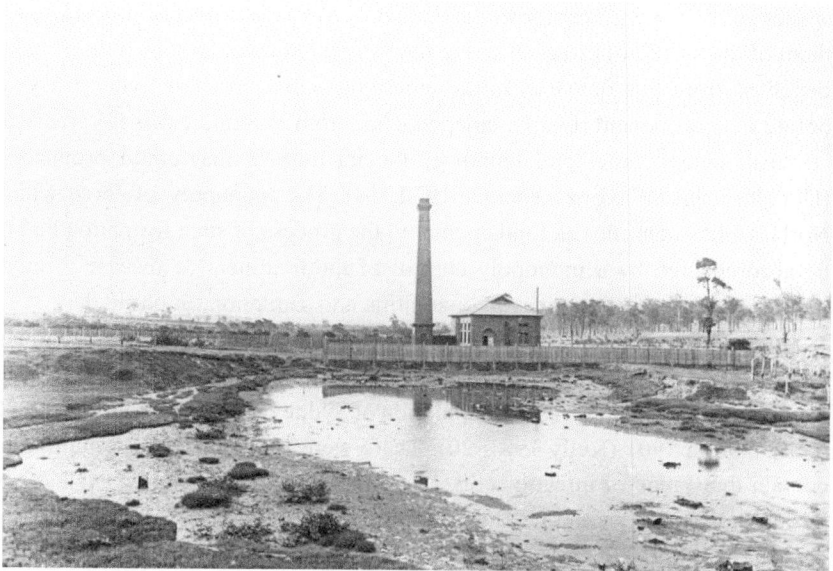

Figure 4 Botany Sewerage Farm [A-00069843]. Image courtesy: Sydney Water Photograph Collection at City of Sydney Archives.

The city was also where people were most likely to get sick with diseases (Curson et al. 1989, 87). As Arthur Payne and Captain Dudley learnt the hard way, it was where they were most likely to be infected with plague (Ashburton-Thompson 1900b, 1860–61). Most of the cases were visitors to the city who actually lived in the suburbs and had commuted in to work, for business or leisure (Ashburton-Thompson 1906, 540). Something had to be done. Notwithstanding Sydney's expansion and the growth of a civic centre, the apprehension of disease haunted the city like a perceived miasma. It countered the calculability of ordered violence of the state with its own incalculable dread. People could not interact in the city without fearing that someone or other might harbour the inconspicuous germs that would cause them harm. The New South Wales government was compelled to increase its administrative reach and efficiency – and pacify public space – by other means beside the constabulary: public health.

4.1 Demand for Public Health

In this historical moment, Sydneysiders were not satisfied with the monopoly of force established by the creation of the police force. They still felt threatened and disgusted by these urban spaces, which the great flight from and avoidance of the city attests to. Another power was called upon to pacify shared urban spaces and free them from the threat of disease as well as violence, indeed, to rid them of the surfeit of affect. And the newly formed institution of public health benefited from this demand. In the emerging social order of Sydney, a year before Federation and relative independence from Britain, it was necessary to establish a new order and empower the institutions that could produce it (Douglas 1966, 37; Enzensberger 1972, 14). The monopoly of force which Norbert Elias identifies as fundamental to the process of state formation had to be accompanied by a monopoly control of the treatment of disease through public health and its practices of quarantine and sanitation, in particular.

Shirley Fitzgerald identifies a particular intransigence and reluctance to act on matters of public health in the Colony of New South Wales in the latter half of the nineteenth century, as the population of Sydney grew from 12,000 in 1830 to 496,000 in 1901 (Kelly 1981, 20). There were very few laws attempting to contain the spread of infectious disease on land, addressed almost exclusively through maritime quarantine laws. 'It might be then argued that no amount of pressure was likely to move the inept New South Wales legislature into action,' she argues (Fitzgerald 1987, 100). But the pressure did come, first with the smallpox epidemic in 1881–82 and then in a dramatic fashion with the emotional response to the first plague outbreak in 1900.

Spurred by the scarlet fever outbreak of 1875–76, the colonial authority established a central Board of Health (Curson 1985, 7). Following the public's strong emotional response to the 1881–82 smallpox epidemic, the government passed additional legislation in 1882 so the Board could operate as an independent Statutory Authority under the 1882 Infectious Diseases Supervision Act, which also required compulsory notification of infectious disease from medical practitioners and householders, and developed rules and guidelines governing segregation, quarantine, management, and prevention of infectious disease. In Australia each colony, and later state, had its own board of health with central authority (Echenberg 2007, 425).

In 1896 the New South Wales government became the last colony in Australia to pass a Public Health Act. The Act formally extended the powers of the New South Wales Board of Health, giving it unprecedented authority for control of populations of people and animals and intervention across New South Wales (Cummins 2003, 92; Fitzgerald 1987, 88). Empowered by this mandate, the board was prepared for an unprecedented response to the plague. It was notified as people in surrounding countries fell sick, and when the plague was reported in Nouméa in December 1899, it implemented measures to detect and kill rats aboard ships as they docked at port (Thearle et al. 1994, 23). This readiness to respond was reflected in the board's involvement in each of the three main forms of institutional effort to contain and eradicate the plague: the campaign to exterminate rats, the quarantining of patients and contacts in the Maritime Quarantine Station at North Head, and the isolating and cleansing of areas and households throughout the city as well as maritime and urban fumigation.

The board's Chief Medical Officer Dr John Ashburton-Thompson was a perceptive leader who achieved a measure of global fame for his response to the plague in Sydney. Having trained in general practice and public health in England he followed developments in medical science from his post in Sydney, where he administered one of the most progressive responses to plague in the British Empire, informed by the latest research in the new science of bacteriology. Doctors were starting to become better acquainted with the emerging science, and more confident that the laboratory rather than the clinic was the proper diagnostic site. Unfortunately for Dudley and 101 other Sydneysiders, however, while filling one lacuna in medical knowledge, the development of new diagnostic methods destabilised understandings of control of infectious disease without resolving all questions of prevention and treatment. The discourses that were produced in response to this uncertainty used the symbol of dirt to authorise their perspectives and proposed solutions. Since dirt had the power to endanger order, it had to be cleaned up (Douglas 1966, 35).

4.2 Debate over Quarantine

There was substantive disagreement between the Ashburton-Thompson and the New South Wales government about whether the plague was communicated from person to person. By contrast with highly contagious diseases like the pneumonic form of the plague or smallpox, Ashburton-Thompson argued that only the bubonic and septicaemic forms of plague were present in Sydney, and that they would therefore not be transmitted by sputum exchanged in interactions between people, the '[p]lague as seen at Sydney during the outbreak under notice was not "catching"' (Ashburton-Thompson 1900b, 33). Notwithstanding his relatively informed position, he directed the Board to not quarantine contacts or homes of plague victims, unless they were so irresponsible that their premises might harbour rats and fleas, that is, if their homes were 'overcrowded and filthy, and presumably a source of infection' (Ashburton-Thompson 1900b, 16). Only the presence of the ambiguously defined 'filth' which must harbour rats was a pretext for intervention. It was his view instead that the real threat to people was posed by the population of infected rats who hosted the infection. Rats and any contaminated materials which had come into contact with the sick were targeted as disgust objects during this outbreak.

The parliament of the colony of New South Wales debated the question of whether quarantine of Dudley's contacts had been necessary. In June, Governor William Lyne recalled that he was advised by Ashburton-Thompson not to do so, whom he quoted, '[i]f you read the history of the plague, wherever it has taken place, you will find that in two months from the present time you will probably have 100 patients a day, and you, therefore, cannot quarantine the patients and the contacts'. Lyne later said he responded that 'if that is the decision of the Board of Health, I am going to quarantine the patients and the contacts, too and when it gets beyond me, then I can say I am beaten but not before' (New South Wales Parliament 1900a, 109). People who had been in contact with the sick were going to be suspect.

Ashburton-Thompson recognised that public fear of contacts was caused by association of the plague with other diseases, particularly with the pneumatic form of the plague, which can be transmitted by sputum passed in interactions between people. During and after the epidemic Ashburton-Thompson stated publicly that the principal form of the plague present in Sydney was bubonic, with only seventeen cases recorded of the septicaemic form. Neither of these two forms of plague was contagious, communicated from person to person (Ashburton-Thompson 1900b, 7). For this reason, Ashburton-Thompson advocated a more moderate approach, arguing strongly that public fear and government pressure ought to yield to the advice of medical authorities – which recommended against quarantining contacts. The 'fears and fancies which preoccupy the mind of the general public on such occasions, and the dicta of those among them who rely for guidance on common sense, cause confusion, sap confidence, favour panic, and pave the way for disaster' (Ashburton-Thompson 1900b, 43). Other doctors agreed, with one complaining that by quarantining contacts the Government 'has pursued a course which cannot fail to foster and humour the panic of the excessively ignorant public' (Sydney Morning Herald 1900b, 8). A lack of established medical knowledge resulted in profound division.

While there was some disagreement with the New South Wales government about whether the quarantine of contacts was necessary, it produced different typologies of contacts to justify more coercive orders. The Board used its executive authority to forcibly remove resistant contacts multiple times, including sixty guests of two hotels in the city (Echenberg 2007, 251). Ashburton-Thompson defined contacts as either people who had contact with plague rats in the previous five days, who had contact with a person who had the septicaemic case of plague, or who had contact with someone who was ill with or dead from plague. In some cases it also meant anyone who shared a household with someone who had become sick, who had to be evacuated while their home was sanitised (Ashburton-Thompson 1901, 166). He distinguished these 'contacts' from people who had been in close quarters with someone who merely suffered bubonic plague.

Some contacts were removed to the Quarantine Station. Others found themselves locked in their homes, their workplaces, or their suburbs, if these spaces were designated as infected and closed by the authorities. On Friday, March 9, the *Sydney Morning Herald* reported the case of Wesley Stratford, an eight-year-old boy admitted to the Hospital for Sick Children in Glebe with a wound to his knee. The boy had apparently patted a dog which was suspected of having the plague. Later blood tests examined under a microscope revealed the plague bacillus. He was immediately taken to quarantine, and his house was isolated for cleaning. According to this report, while the Board of Health opposed quarantining the entire hospital, the Premier William Lyon, 'consistently with the view he had previously enunciated', issued instructions for all forty-six patients and staff (including the dispenser and the gardener) to be 'peremptorily "shut in"' through quarantine, and for the hospital to be rigorously cleansed and disinfected (Sydney Morning Herald 1900c, 3). Fortunately for the 'inmates' their imprisonment did not last too long. After a special meeting of the Board of Health the hospital staff and patients were offered vaccination with Haffkine's prophylactic and eventually released from quarantine. This backflip over quarantine illustrates the way changing medical evaluations of the risk influenced people's perception of the threat and their changing responses.

Structures of confinement like quarantine differentiated bodies and regulated the traffic of them through social space to keep it functioning effectively (Foucault 1975, 22–38; Waldby 1996, 89). Michael Foucault situates this symbolic effort to contain the body in relation to the history of the state. In *Discipline and Punish: The Birth of the Prison*, he identifies a transformation: from a sovereign power with the right to take the life of its subjects, to a disciplinary power, with the right to administer, manage, and, if necessary, confine its population. These strategies subjugated bodies and controlled groups with what Foucault terms 'biopower', internalising the operations of power in the body under the guise of improving the health of the individual and the population (Foucault 1977, 137–45). In Sydney this effort to contain and regulate the dangerous potential of the body produced what historian Alison Bashford refers to as 'boundaries of rule' or spaces of public health across the city (Bashford 2004, 1).

For Douglas, '[a] polluting person is always in the wrong. He has developed some wrong condition or simply crossed some line which should not have been crossed and his displacement unleashes danger on someone' (Douglas 1966, 113). The expression of disgust aims to protect the self from this perceived threat by establishing distance, it is spatial. The concept is closely linked to other spatial actions of aversion, which stems from the Latin *avertere*, to turn away, and abjection, from *abjacere*, to cast out or reject. Psychoanalytic theorist Julia Kristeva's concept of the abject is correspondingly one of a substance that has crossed a boundary, which we loathe, fear, and repulse with great ferocity. The volatility of this substance, its ambiguous status between inside and outside of the body, of the home, of the city, reveals the fragility of these boundaries and results in fierce efforts to reinforce it to protect identity (Kristeva 1982, 18). According to Kristeva, the process of exclusion of the abject also produces the boundaries of the self (Kristeva 1982, 73). The spatial qualities of disgust as a means of creating distance or producing the boundaries of identity were apparent in the public health interventions of 1900, which pushed out things and people defined as abject to produce the boundaries of a pacified city, colony, and territory.

4.3 Pure Order

Once they quarantined a plague case, the Board of Health closed that house or workplace for cleaning for up to eight days (Ashburton-Thompson 1900b, 78). A Notice to Cleanse and Disinfect issued under the Public Health Act made the householder themselves responsible for cleansing, disinfecting, or destroying certain items on their premises or paying the department to do so (Ashburton-Thompson 1900b, 80). If there was a cluster of cases, it closed the streets, and sometimes the suburb. From March 23rd to July 17th the programme closed successive portions of the city to traffic (Ashburton-Thompson 1900b, 18). Over several weeks people were unable to enter or leave parts of Sydney like Darling Harbour. While isolated for cleaning, the suburb was cut off from the city like a rotten limb. After the results of the Plague Department of Sydney City Municipal Council were deemed inadequate, the New South Wales Government took over the cleaning operation, citing the apprehension and aversion of the city by the public (Sydney Morning Herald 1900a, 9).

Yet on March 23rd, when architect George McCredie took leadership of the plague cleaning team, he immediately encountered several problems (Kelly 1981, 6, 14). First, many of the people stuck in parts of the city that had been quarantined were complaining of hunger. Some of them did not have a place to stay, as they had been prevented from returning home when quarantine was suddenly imposed. He organised some food from the restaurants in the area, and even found accommodation for the unlucky people who were stuck. His second problem of appointing inspectors and arranging housing for workmen was harder to solve. He could not find staff. In a report to the Premier of New South Wales he said, 'I applied to men I knew to be competent to take the responsible positions, but met with so many refusals, although offered 20s. per day, that it seemed as though the difficulties would be insuperable. Very few would take the risk to which they considered they would be exposed by accepting employment in the very hotbed of the plague' (New South Wales Parliament 1900a, 110). If contacts could spread the plague, and if suspicious bodies or places could potentially harbour microbes, any intimacy with people or homes suspected of disease was to be strictly avoided. Eventually McCredie found some staff by applying to the Board of Health, the Board of Works, and the Labour Bureau. He also recruited some of the quarantined men who suddenly found themselves stranded and unemployed, paying them 8s. a day to clean everything within the barriers. Over time the fear and disgust people felt at the prospect of sanitation work changed. People even began to deliberately loiter in an area that was scheduled to be quarantined, so they would be forced to stay and could apply for work as incarcerated cleaning crew (New South Wales Parliament 1900a, 111).

In Ashburton-Thompson's words, McCredie's job was to sublimate '[d]arkness, dampness, filth, and bad construction of dwellings' across Sydney (Ashburton-Thompson 1900b, 47). Once the cleaning team identified a suspect building, they had a long list of actions to perform. First the ceilings, walls, cellars, and basement all had to be washed in lime. Exposed woodwork and covered floors had to be scrubbed with carbolic water; any stone or brick floors had to be saturated. Drains, pipes, sinks, and water closets were flushed with hot water and then a mixture of the lime and carbolic acid. Furniture, machinery, and merchandise had to be moved so the cleaning team could access the floors and walls, even in businesses or warehouses. Any waste material, including manure or human waste, was removed.

But Sydney's transition to chemical modernity did not go smoothly. To be targeted by the cleaning operation could be inconvenient, embarrassing, or even ruinous. Adding to McCredie's problems, some people wrote letters or made statements trying to prevent his team from visiting their property altogether. In a speech to parliament, Sir William Lyne claimed the manager of a large shipping company said to McCredie, '"[k]eep down there at the bottom of the stairs; anything you have to say to me must be said from there". That was the state of the public feeling of the time', he said (New South Wales Parliament 1900b, 113).

In July, Louis Blackwell, the City of Sydney council's Inspector of Nuisances and Special Officer of their Plague Department, wrote to the Town Clerk to notify him that cleaning crews had destroyed the toilets, floorboards, stair-cases, and other fittings in several houses in Washington Lane (see Figure 5)

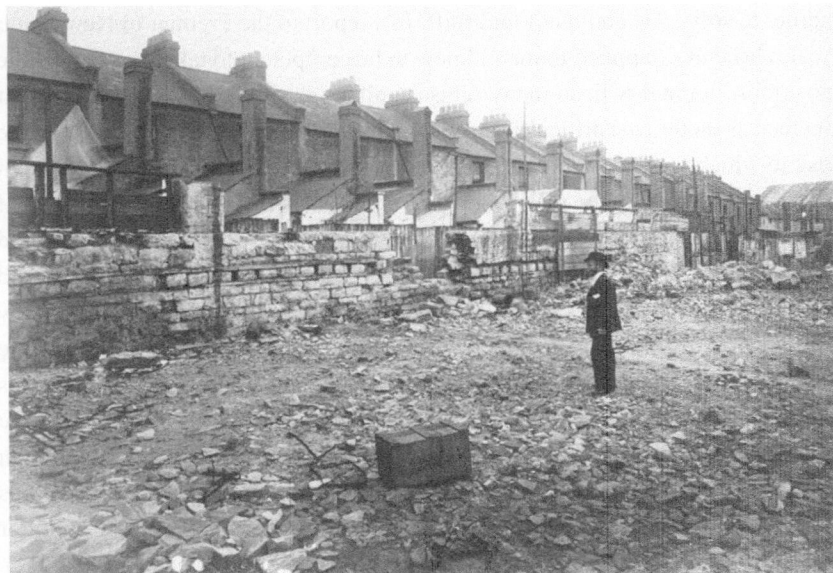

Figure 5 Brick Terrace Housing in Washington Street Sydney [A-00036166]. City of Sydney Demolition Books, 1900. Image courtesy: City of Sydney Archives.

(Town Clerk's Correspondence Folders 17th July 1900a). One report to the New South Wales parliament accused some of the men in McCredie's cleaning team of acting like 'pirates'.

> They went and put chloride of lime in pianos, and diluted sulphuric acid on glass, and they did all they could to prevent this scourge spreading. A very respected lady in my electorate had her doorstep removed. I do not know if the fine susceptibilities of one of the cleaners were wounded by the thought that this might convey to some casual passer-by the seed of the disease; but, at any rate, he took it away . . . all of this has brought about a very large number of complaints, accompanied by a very natural irritation by the people who were quarantined. (New South Wales Parliament 1900a, 214)

The team had done even more damage to a few houses in Bathurst Street, he added, leaving a gushing leak from a broken water pipe and drain 'freely emitting sewer gases'. In July the Town Clerk Robert McAnderson wrote to the under-secretary for trade and finance, requesting better supervision of cleansing staff and accusing them of the 'wanton destruction of property' (Town Clerk's Correspondence Folders 17th July 1900a). In parliament, opposition leader Mr Reid reported that the sight of an allegedly plague infected rat at a building in Haymarket resulted in extreme overreaction, as police evacuated the building and had the cleaning team burn its entire

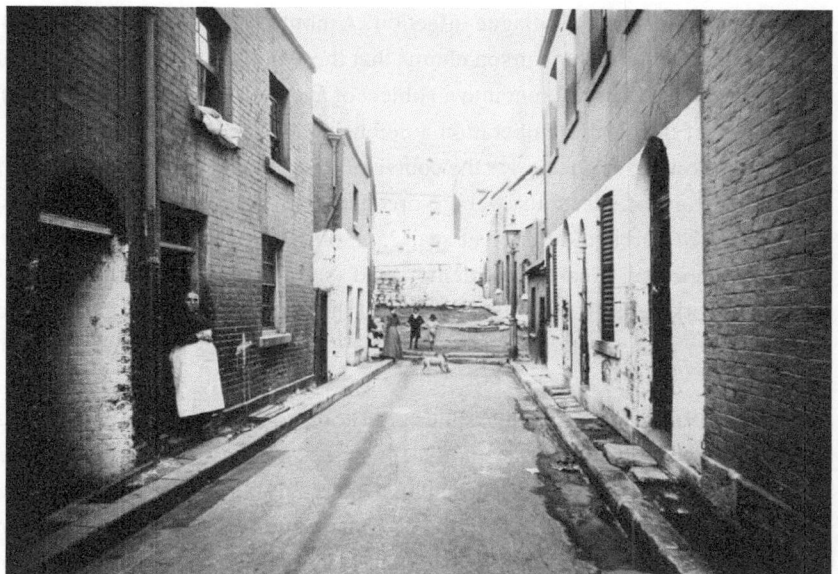

Figure 6 Terrace houses in Bates Lane Sydney [A-00036120], City of Sydney
Demolition Books, 1900. Image courtesy: City of Sydney Archives.

contents. Unable to verify the report of the rat, all the Board of Health could do
was to apologise (New South Wales Parliament 1900a, 81–3). Complaints
were so numerous that McCredie had to meticulously document his operations
by taking photographs, in case he needed future evidence of the state of
disrepair of the targeted homes. These photographs have become part of the
City of Sydney 'Demolition Books' (see Figure 6) and state government
archives.

The programme of housing demolition was the first of its kind under the
Public Health Act in Sydney. Throughout Moore Park, Darling Harbour, and the
Rocks, 425 'filthy and overcrowded' buildings were condemned and 146 were
demolished, 'presumably a source of infection' (Ashburton-Thompson 1900b,
16; Mayne 1993, 103). In June, the Town Clerk of the Sydney City Council
applied to the Inspector of Nuisances for condemnation of a 'very suspicious'
building which looked like an 'Oyster Saloon' at 191 Elizabeth Street. Inside
there were fourteen or fifteen 'badly lighted and ventilated bedrooms with
double beds in every instance' which appeared to be used for 'immoral pur-
poses' (Town Clerk's Correspondence Folders 27th July 1900d). The 'notorious
brothel' was referred for condemnation.

Even the buildings left standing had their problems, becoming symbolic of
moral degeneracy. A small placard was affixed to one which stated that it had

been officially cleansed of plague infection (Ashburton-Thompson 1900b, 80). Medical geographer Peter Curson claims that these notices became a 'badge of shame' and made their referent into an object of aversion (Curson 1985, 153–5). By the end of the cleaning operation a defensive McCredie reported to parliament the following metrics: over the course of four months a total of 4,000 staff had 52,030 tons of silt and sewerage dredged from the front of the wharves; 28,455 tons of garbage dumped at sea; 25,430 tons of garbage burned; 3,808 premises inspected, cleansed or demolished (see Figure 7); 17,000 rats destroyed by workmen; 27,548 rats destroyed at the rat depot for a fee; 1,423 dead animals taken from the harbour and burnt (New South Wales Parliament 1900b, 112).

For the usually phlegmatic Ashburton-Thompson, this population of rats around the decaying structures and dark recesses of the harbourside wharves and inner-city terraces was a particularly execrable disgust object, 'for dirt, decay, darkness and filth . . . favour the presence of rats' (Ashburton-Thompson 1900b, 47). He urged a 'crusade against rats', making it a pillar of his sanitation programme, officiated with missionary zeal by individuals and institutions alike (Ashburton-Thompson 1900b, 15–16). Historian Myron Echenberg has noted that this focus on 'vector control' was central to the response in Sydney, which

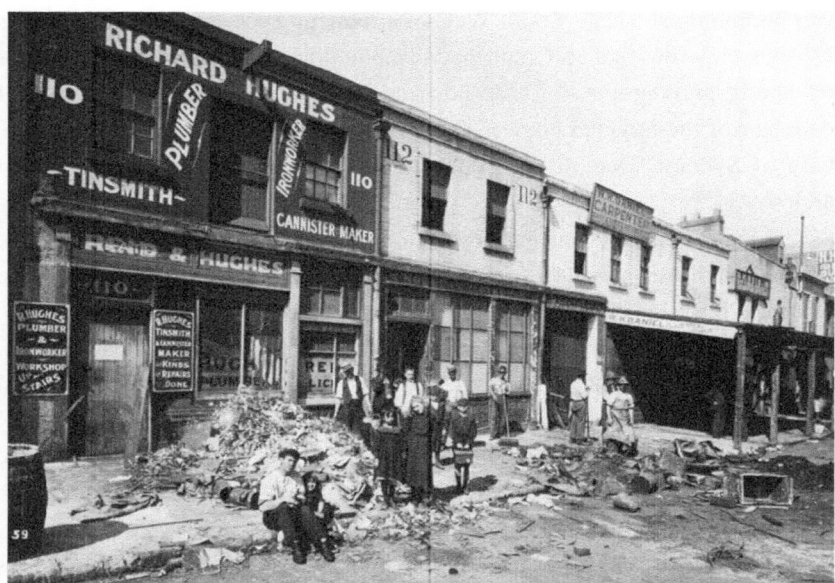

Figure 7 Views taken during Cleansing Operations, Kent Street, Sydney, 1900, Vol. I. Under the supervision of Mr George McCredie, NSW. 1900. Image courtesy: Collections of the State Library of New South Wales.

Echenberg contends was one of the more progressive and successful efforts to contain plague worldwide (Echenberg 2002, 444; Echenberg 2007, 250, 264). Yet the sanitation campaign was not simply a response to the threat of pollution and an effort to transform rats into vanquished disgust objects. It was an act of institutional aversion and ritual purification intended to build confidence in the new order, particularly in the institutional authorities which governed that order in time for the 1901 Federation.

4.4 Urban Change and State Formation

The discursive strategy which mobilised disgust and fear was successful. People were affected enough to embrace change. The acceptance and demand for the intervention of public health is particular to the status of Sydney as a society looking to redeem its deviant colonial past and environment for the safety of the British settler population. The plague was an historic opportunity to cast out anything abject, anything that was considered incompatible with the creation of an identity as citizens of the new nation of Australia. If the abject produces the borders of our being through this act of expulsion, to be a proper citizen of the new Federation, it was necessary to collaborate in the purgation of the city and cast out people and objects that were regarded as inimical to health (Kristeva 1982, 101).

The level of buy-in during the 1900 outbreak in Sydney was quite distinct from other responses to the plague throughout the British Empire. In India, by contrast, the incredibly coercive public health response of the colonial rulers was heavily resisted across multiple classes, as historian David Arnold has shown. There was a much greater focus on the body of the colonial subject, which was a presumed vector of disease, than on rats (Arnold 1982, 61). The British attempted to figure the Indian colonial subjects themselves as disgust objects. This resulted in a coercive set of policies adopted by colonial author-ities in towns and cities to protect the health of the colonisers by controlling the bodies of Indian sex workers, servants, soldiers, plantation labourers deemed a threat to the British. The clash between the practices of public health and local cultural practices resulted in intense resistance in cities such as Bombay, Pune, Karachi, and Calcutta where public health ignored notions of caste and religion and as obstacles to sanitary reform (Arnold 1982, 58–9). For example, the medical practice of inspecting women's lymph nodes for physical symptoms of buboes was considered tantamount to sexual molestation (Arnold 1982, 64). Even though European medical ideas and practices were becoming more acceptable to the educated Indian middle class, there was a profound resentment among these groups towards the public health policies of segregation and hospitalisation, which manifested in an 'assumption of British self-interest and spite' and a belief in their readiness to sacrifice Indians to preserve British power (Arnold 1982, 61, 76).

When the emotional reaction, or 'spirit of discontent', was too strong, the government gave up on the policy, as they considered emotive political discontent more dangerous than disease (Arnold 1982, 81). Indeed by 1907 Ashburton-Thompson himself was advising the Indian Plague Commission and authorities to focus their efforts on 'the exclusion of rats from occupied buildings in cities' which he argued was 'the only measure which can permanently diminish the susceptibility of India to plague' (Ashburton-Thompson 1907a, 1771). The more coercive aspects of public health policy were abandoned in favour of more voluntary measures or those promoted by trusted agencies. Eventually British colonial authorities realised that inviting cooperation of local leaders was preferable to mass resistance and unchecked spread of plague (Arnold 1982, 86). The situation in the British colonies in India can be strongly contrasted with that of the colony of New South Wales, where the public health measures were either energetically demanded or only passively resisted. As Ashburton-Thompson proudly if erroneously proclaimed, in Sydney the population was 'not merely wholly white, of English extraction and speech, and fully civilised, but intelligent, instructed, and orderly, accustomed to direction and amenable to it' (Ashburton-Thompson 1906, 538).

5 'A Maze of Contradictory Observations': Medical Eclecticism and Changing Understandings of Disease Causation

Ashburton-Thompson's fervent desire to understand the complex ecology of the plague was in part due to a belief that the colony of New South Wales should be distinguished from the British colonies of India and Hong Kong. Some practitioners had hypothesised that plague was prevalent in India because it was contracted by locals who walked barefoot through the soil infested with plague bacillus. For Ashburton-Thompson, the cultural practices of Sydneysiders negated this thesis, as 'the inhabitants of Sydney no more go barefoot than do the inhabitants of London' (Ashburton-Thompson 1901, 166). Sydney was not like the other colonies, it was in his view, much more 'civilised'.

When an epidemic of plague possibly originating in the Himalayas spread from China to Hong Kong in 1893, teams of competing French and Japanese bacteriologists stationed in Hong Kong intensified their efforts to identify the agent of the disease. By July 1894, Dr Alexander Yersin and Dr Shiba Saburo Kitasato had both identified bacteria in the tissues of rats and people infected with the plague. But Yersin was the first to file a report with the Academy of

Sciences in France, naming the bacillus that caused the plague *Pasteurella pestis* (Thearle et al. 1994, 8; Watts 1997, 5; Yersin and Treille 1894). In 1971 this bacillus was called *Yersinia pestis* and categorised in a genus called Yersinia, which includes the *Yersinia enterocolitica* that infected me during the revising of this Element (Collins 1996; Savin et al. 2019, 1). Yet identification of the bacteria did not stop infected rats making their way on board the thousands of boats entering and leaving Hong Kong harbour, a crucial British Empire trade node. By 1900 the plague had docked at ports all over the world, with the pandemic extending from Noumea to San Francisco, Glasgow to Sydney.

While researching a particularly virulent outbreak of plague in India in 1896, French epidemiologist Dr Paul-Lewis Simond published a theory that the most likely vector of plague transmission between rats and people was the flea (Ashmead 1901, 13; Simond et al. 1901, 36–7; Watts 1997, 5). In an article published on the anniversary of his initial theory, his nephew argued that Simond's theory was received with scepticism and derision from many of his colleagues, particularly European epidemiologists. An article in *Nature* published in 1907 confirms that only with experimentation by scientists Gauthier and Raybaud in Marseilles in 1902 was it first established that plague could infect fleas and that these fleas could bite people (Anon 1907). The same article validates these experiments with reference to Ashburton-Thompson's pioneering epidemiological work in Sydney which showed the role of the flea to be the most likely explanation for how plague was transmitted from rats to people, proving the influence of his research in the international medical community at that time. The article also refers to Sydney bacteriologist Frank Tidswell's 1903 experiments to determine the species of flea responsible for transmission. However even at this point there was still some questions unanswered in 'the exact method by which the bacilli are conveyed; why so many other investigators have failed in similar experiments, and whether rats transmit the disease in any other way' (Anon 1907, 60).

Dr Ashburton-Thompson was indeed one of very few public health officials in the world who earnestly investigated Simond's theory, believing that there must be some intermediary to transmit plague from rat to humans (Ashburton-Thompson 1900a, 4; Ashburton-Thompson 1900b, 70). Throughout the first outbreak he was cautious in his approach, but gradually collected data to test the theory that plague was spread by rats (Ashburton-Thompson 1900a, 5). In addition, he produced a series of reports after each outbreak which attempted to establish the ecology of disease transmission and explored Simond's hypothesis. He authored publications in *The Lancet*, *The Journal of Hygiene*, and the *St Louis Medical and Surgical Journal* (Ashburton-Thompson 1901; Ashburton-Thompson 1903; Ashburton-Thompson 1904; Ashburton-Thompson 1907b).

In a report published in *The Journal of Hygiene* in 1901, he suggested that there must be two hosts of the disease for an individual to become infected – the rat and a 'suctorial parasite'.

In a 1903 article in *The Lancet* Ashburton-Thompson endorsed Simond's hypothesis as the most likely, without concluding it had been proven (Ashburton-Thompson 1903, 1092). In his 1907 report in *The Lancet*, he clarified that there was insufficient evidence to determine the role of the flea in the complex ecology of the plague until 1905. But only after years of collecting data in each outbreak did he finally conclude with a publication in *The Lancet* in 1907:

> The way in which plague spreads is one and the same everywhere . . . Plague epizootic in the rat is the essential factor in the diffusion of this disease and in the production of its epidemic form, but the infection of the plague rat cannot be commonly communicated to man except with the help of an intermediary. The efficient intermediary is the flea, which infests the rat and occasionally attacks man after its proper host has died. (Ashburton-Thompson 1907b, 1104)

Unfortunately, many of Ashburton-Thompson's colleagues were less progressive and dismissed his supposition. An editorial note concluded that the 'experimental data presented in these publications do not tend to support Simond's hypothesis' (Ashburton-Thompson 1901, 162–3). Simond's hypothesis was confirmed in 1903 by Gauthier and Raybaud in Marseilles, but only following the research by the English Commission in India were mechanisms of plague transmission generally accepted in the scientific community in 1906 (Simond et al. 1998, 103).

Ashburton-Thompson's research in Sydney played a pivotal role in the acceptance of Simond's theory. By 1907 his research was being cited retrospectively in *Nature* (Anon 1907). While Ashburton-Thompson quickly began to explore potential transmission pathways, at the time of the first outbreak of the plague he had to respond without the benefit of this knowledge, recognising only that he needed more evidence. Indeed, he was not even decisively sure himself until November 1900 that the plague was not communicated by the sick (Ashburton-Thompson 1907a, 1770). Ideas about disease transmission were confused.

For the duration of the first outbreak in 1900, even Ashburton-Thompson was uncertain

> whether the rat infected man, or man the rat, and whether both did not acquire the disease independently of each other from some source which was common to both. In the meantime this clue had been taken in hand at Sydney, and

an attempt had been made to follow it through the maze which apparently contradictory observations had gradually woven. (Ashburton-Thompson 1907b, 1104–5)

A 1901 article in the *St Louis Medical and Surgical Journal* based on Ashburton-Thompson's 1900 report continued to speculate as to whether the excreta or mucous of the rat could transmit the plague, particularly through the contamination of food, though he admitted that man 'rarely if ever gets the disease by ingestion' (Ashmead 1901, 12–13). Simond et al. concur that one of the reasons the international medical community was resistant to the theory of the role of the flea in transmission of the plague was because they were 'not ready to accept that any biting insect could act as a vector for disease; instead most clinicians believed that 'miasmas' formed the main transmission path for infectious diseases' (Simond et al. 1998, 103).

While beginning to learn about the new science of bacteriology, medical practitioners adopted what Fitzgerald describes as an 'eclectic view of disease transmission, preferring whatever explanation seemed to best suit the occasion' (Fitzgerald 1987, 76). By late April in the year of the first plague outbreak, the *Sydney Morning Herald* was reporting '[e]ven professional medical men were at sea in many instances as regarded knowledge of how the trouble was propagated' (Sydney Morning Herald 1900j, 10). Notwithstanding this nascent medical knowledge and ongoing investigation, odours were still considered a threat in 1900. Historian Shirley Fitzgerald claims that many medical practitioners in Sydney continued to believe in the miasmatic theories of disease causation, which is to say, that disease was spread by noxious vapours or miasma and could be indicated by a bad smell, perhaps coming from rubbish or human waste. Widely understood as a 'corruption and infection of the air', miasma was considered bad air, recognisable by odour, that could be generated by evaporation from marshes, inauspicious alignment of the stars, smoke from erupting volcanos or the stench of any form of decay (Ashmead 1901, 13; Simond et al. 1901, 36–7; Watts 1997, 5).

Public perception of odours did not change with transformation in medical knowledge. Indeed, Jenner argues that there were 'substantial continuities in attitudes' as 'bad smells continued to generate considerable sanitary anxiety'. Residents could sense for themselves the strange smells that emanated from threatening sites across the city, be they rubbish dumps, cemeteries, slums, or factories using toxic chemicals. They also recognised that people living or working at these sites were often sick. Either smell was the miasma that made you sick, or it provoked an affective reaction that indicated something that could threaten you, such as the plague. Jenner argued that there was an intertwining of bacteriological and miasmatic theories of disease causation, which he described as a 'sanitary-bacteriological synthesis' (Jenner 2011, 346). In the Hippocratic framework, where air has a direct physical effect on the body that inhales, foul smells were not just disgusting, but abject and poisonous sources of disease. By contrast, fresh or perfumed air was considered therapeutic. Thus in 1900 Sydney there was a resolute demand for fumigation, the desire to literally breathe in the perception of cleanliness.

6 Transforming the Atmosphere

The notion that odours may also have symbolic value is not without its complexity, as pointed out by anthropologist Alfred Gell (Gell 1975). While an unpleasant odour may have significance, it does not belong to a sign system in the same way that linguistic terms like dirt and filth do. But odours always indicate a referent object and when they are sensed by a subject within a particular context they also work as symbols. As Lewis argues, '[w]e do not discover the meaning of a certain smell by distinguishing it from other smells (we have no independent means of codifying these distinctions) but by distinguishing contexts within which particular smells have typical value' (Lewis 1977, 27).

In this case the relevant context is Sydney's liminal status between British colony and independent city. As historian Alecia Simmonds argues, the Australian history of smell needs to be distinguished from the existing historiography of smell (Simmonds 2019, 236). In the Australian context, women like Mrs Dudley had a role to play in a process of sanitary reform that was more cooperative, based on an idea of creating a post-colonial subject who would be entitled to the rights of citizens in the new nation. Odours also drew boundaries between subjects who were to be become citizens – 'whites', in Ashburton-Thompson's terminology – and those who were not from European backgrounds or who were from class backgrounds that undermined the social mobility of the city.

In 1902 the medical officer of the local government board of England, Bruce Low, published a report on the diffusion of the third pandemic of the plague across the colonies of the British Empire between 1898 and 1901. He detailed a range of responses from highly coercive measures that met with strong local resistance in cities across India, to public health interventions with considerable local acceptance such as in New South Wales. But Low was surprised by the conditions in Sydney. He had assumed settler colonial societies would not share the sanitation problems of established European cities like Paris or London (Reinarz 2014, 196–7). This was not the case, however. At the end of the nineteenth century in New Zealand, Dunedin's harbour was nicknamed 'Stinkapool' due to the odours produced by its unmanaged problems of sewerage, drainage, and waste (Reinarz 2014, 196–7). In Low's report, Sydney did not fare much better. 'Sydney, of all Australian towns, was the dirtiest,' he said. 'The streets in the lower part of the town were said to be seldom clear of refuse of hide and wool scourings, which under the conditions of humid atmosphere, gave off emanations of a most unsavoury sort' (Low 1902, 394).

6.1 Noxious Trades

There was, of course, an ongoing tension between these symbolic beliefs about odour being a cause of disease and odours as a representation or index of a polluting substance that could cause ill health. An aversion to bad odours was not simply emotional. Toxic or hazardous sites could be poisonous, and at the turn of the century, the barometer of their potential potency, even within legal contexts, was their smell. Indeed, the term 'noxious trade' was applied to industrial activities which stank, rather than those which were polluting or toxic to health (Fitzgerald 1987, 88). In his annual report for 1899, the Inspector of Nuisances went to court to report two breaches of the Noxious Trades Act for 'fat melting' and to force the businesses to close (Baker 1900). Across the city there were slaughterhouses, butchers, piggeries, gluemakers, poultry farms, fellmongers, bone mills, tanneries, and rope manufacturers working with pungent poisons like lead, mercury, and arsenic that caused occupational hazards and illness. The *Votes and Proceedings of the Legislative Assembly* in 1900 are replete with reports of factories issuing noxious and offensive vapours. One report admonished soup driers, pig keepers, and bone grinders for consistently allowing the noxious vapours generated by their trades to offend the local community. Even the Mayor of Alexandria himself had been summoned to court for offending his own nuisance by-laws (Fitzgerald 1987, 88, 90). The high volume of complaints eventually resulted in the Royal Commission on Noxious and Offensive Trades in 1882 (New South Wales 1883).

A corollary process of urban reform was entrusted to the institution of public health that emerged in the 1880s. It focused on eliminating multiple sources of bad smells with improvements to the network of drains and sewers, as well as regulation of household waste (including effluent), prevention of nuisances like household odours, and location of noxious trades which used poisonous chemicals like lead and arsenic. By 1886, the power of municipal councils to pass by-laws to control industries gazetted as noxious was repealed. This power was transferred to the central government when the Noxious Trades and Cattle Slaughtering Act of 1886 gave the Board of Health jurisdiction over municipal regulation of noxious trades, which left councils as mere administrators of the Board's decisions (Fitzgerald 1987, 93).

6.2 Desire for a New Sensory Order

Bad odours and their sources had to be cleaned up. Yet as Kristeva argues, the exclusion of waste to create the boundaries of a clean person or place is never entirely straightforward. During McCredie's cleaning campaign, a long debate raged in the papers about the relocation or eradication of Sydney's rubbish dumps, which were consistently associated with abject odours. A landfill at Moore Park was particularly reviled after a father and his three children all contracted the plague in their reportedly flea-infested household and died. The children played there, while their father was one of the local scavengers (Echenberg 2007, 248). *The Truth* ranted, 'this festering bubo on the body of the city should be burnt out with chemicals or with fire' (The Truth 1900a, 1). The Bulletin preferred to represent it as that which must be obliterated to enable the 'civilising' of Sydney, arguing that '[i]n any decently civilised city garbage isn't "tipped", nor buried, nor thrown in a river or harbour, nor even dropped into the sea so that a great part of it may wash up again on the shoes along 100 miles of coast. It is utterly destroyed by fire' (The Bulletin 1900b, 6). The *Sunday Times* reported that the Sydney City Council resisted change, 'the Mayor practically declared last Tuesday that the Mount Rennie refuse heap was a harmless spot, which anyone might visit without inconvenience' (Sunday Times 1900a, 2). However, the medical community seemingly disagreed. Dr Gresswell from the Victorian Board of Health described it as a 'horrible abomination', all the time

> belching forth from its seething mass of tens of thousands of tons of putrefying filth its pestiferous odours, and yielding to the suction exercised by variations of barometric pressure almost every vile germ, in myriads, that lived for the discomfort of man and animal ... Poisonous vapours and gases and disease forming germs are given off into the atmosphere, and these, together with rodents and insect vermin, will never be fairly combated so long as the continuance of this common tip is countenanced in the centre of the population. (Sunday Times 1900a, 2)

The air itself had become a disgust object.

In Sydney in 1900, confusion about whether plague was spread by air and the risk posed by noxious trades made odours a particularly potent trigger of disgust. Odours are fugitives; they escape from their objects (Lewis 1977, 27). Within the social and spatial context of the city, this escapism gave rise to a particularly anxious form of abjection. As Reinarz argues, odours have a unique mobility, they can cross boundaries in a way the other senses cannot, they are easier to share, they are unstoppable (Reinarz 2014, 19). It is also very hard to trace them back to their sources. They are confusing, mysterious (Miller 1997, 66). Odours are dynamic, drifting around as airborne particles. A negative or unpleasant odour also indicates a state of instability, of decay or decomposition, which seems to signify a transformative power, perhaps to heal or to destroy (Reinarz 2014, 8): 'the coming into being and passing away of things, situations, circumstances, which hold our attention vividly while they are present' (Lewis 1977, 28). By implicating the decaying object in the subject, odours can be particularly abject, provoking violent distancing responses. Not only does odour indicate a violent proximity, but it cannot be properly expelled. To smell an odour is to become or incorporate it (Borthwick 2000, 127, 130). It entails contact, dissolves distance. Suddenly you are not separate from the thing that disgusts you. Identity is at risk once the boundaries that produce the self are overcome. Disgust can try to sputter out the unwanted presence, but it cannot succeed. The drive to cast out an odour is impossibly fraught.

Even after George McCredie closed the Moore Park rubbish dump, it continued to cause complaints. McCredie resolved to burn as much rubbish as possible and to dump whatever remained off punts out at sea. This resulted in rubbish washing up on the harbour foreshore at beaches around Sydney, causing complaints from the harbour and beachside councils of Manly, Waverley, and Woollahra. On 3rd April, the Mayor of Sydney received a complaint from the Mayor of Manly asking the council to stem the tide of rubbish from the harbour wharves, as 'a lot of old receipt butts, different kinds of fruit and vegetables, dead fowls and odds and ends' had been collected around the baths or was washing ashore on the Manly and Narrabeen beaches (Fletcher 1900). One resident reportedly wrote to the New South Wales Premier, 'when the north-east winds blow, the effluvium, with its accompanying germs, are carried here and throughout this district'. The writer expressed concern that his 'once clean' corner of the city would now be exposed to the 'dread disease' (Sunday Times 1900c, 7).

On the 25th of March a correspondent for *The Bulletin* complained that people were still entering the rubbish dump to 'scavenge' through the rubbish, heedless of the fact 'the smell was something dreadful' (The Bulletin 1900a, 6). After sand was dumped over the remaining rubbish to try to smother the smell, the surveyor of the Sydney Council reported that trucks simply recommenced dumping rubbish over the top of the sand. 'I have the honour to report that the rubbish carts are at present tipping their contents on the sand recently laid by the Contractors to cover the Moore Park "Private" Tip, and to state that if this is continued the effect of the sand spreading will be neutralised' (Town Clerk's Correspondence Folders 25th July 1900b).

One columnist for the *Sunday Times* argued that 'dirty' places like Redfern and Belmore Park near the centre of the city had been built out of rubbish. While they had not been renowned for disease outbreaks in the past, their 'evil smelling' foundations could have perhaps cultivated seeds of the diseases of plague and typhoid, he argued, which were now ripe for harvest (Sunday Times 1900c, 2). When a cluster of cases appeared around the harbour wharves of Sussex Street in the city, it was determined that all the cases were 'from the class which might be expected to be beset by surroundings conducive to contagion'. All, that is, except a Mr Heaton, who had likely succumbed to the disease after visiting a dry cellar with a pile of dead rodents and, according to his fellow merchants, must have 'breathed pestiferous air', or been infected by fleas that had abandoned the dead rats (Evening News 1900b, 6).

Unsurprisingly, this fear of bad air manifested in a particularly strong aversion to pungent smells. The New South Wales Minister for Works Mr O'Sullivan proposed barrels of pitch and tar be burnt in the streets, to purify the atmosphere. 'The amazingly up-to-date N.S.W. Minister O'Sullivan wants to go back to the devices of the Great Plague of London days and burn barrels of tar in the streets to purify the atmosphere,' mocked an author in *The Bulletin*. 'The next thing will be a naked O'Sullivan with a burning cresset doing the part of Solomon Eagle along Sussex-street. Solomon eagle was another great disinfectant of the old days' (The Bulletin 1900b, 10). The compulsion to purify the atmosphere was experienced so intensely that some parliamentarians proposed the ritual of dance or procession through the streets.

6.3 The Technology of Fumigation

Fumigation did little to prevent plague. Yet the transformation of the odours of organic cargo from ships, horse manure, and leaking sewerage into the acrid odours of sulphur and formalin allayed anxiety and disgust throughout the city of Sydney. When Arthur Payne was diagnosed, the Board of Health fumigated his home. As Ashburton-Thompson recalled,

> Disinfection of the house occupied by the patient was immediately commenced, under superintendence of the Medical Officer of Health for the Metropolitan Combined District (Dr. W. G. Armstrong). Fumigation with burning sulphur was followed by saturation with sublimate solution, at 1 part to 1,000. Articles which could be boiled were so treated on the spot; other articles were removed in canvas bags for disinfection by steam. (Ashburton-Thompson 1900a, 14)

Fumigation restored people's confidence in the indeterminate air they were breathing, masking the signs of new invisible threats with the odours of chemical modernity (Engelmann et al. 2020, 39). As people learnt to fear and repulse odours as indicative of an environment that could host pathogenic germs, they learnt to appreciate the odour of supposedly antimicrobial chemicals. In the nineteenth century, Engelmann and Lynteris argue, fumigation became a technique for the production of a what they refer to as a 'technoscientific utopia' – an efficient way to purify spaces and objects and overcome the costly economic delay of quarantine (Engelmann et al. 2020, 14). For example, in 1830, the Prussian government attempted to fumigate with chlorine every letter, every official Amtsblatt, every file in government possession, as well as garments and belongings of travellers, goods and merchandise in order to ward off the threat of cholera and protect royal authority (Engelmann et al. 2020, 42).

Fumigation was also a means of symbolic purification. Kirmayer and Lévi-Strauss have both argued that rituals involving the use of symbols have a kind of healing effect (Kirmayer 1993, 161–2; Lévi-Strauss 1963, 188, 197–8). Fresh air was considered indicative of good health and a means of soothing and healing sick bodies. In addition to being clean and disinfected, the Local Government Board of England recommended that an isolation hospital for plague patients have a plentiful supply of 'fresh air' (Low 1902, 400). Located on a windswept promontory, the quarantine station at North Head near Sydney's Manly beach was considered an exemplary design which could heal diseases caused by contaminated air.

Back in the centre of the city, citizens and officials also used fumigation to transform the atmosphere around them. At lending libraries across the city, books and magazines were fumigated with formalin, which had a recognisable, but not 'disagreeable', odour (Sunday Times 1900d, 7). Due to anxiety about plague spreading from the city to the regions, the council of the Railway Institute ensured that the library was disinfected weekly, and all incoming books were fumigated by the latest method. These measures were implemented notwithstanding protests that 'there has not been a single case of infectious disease in Sydney traceable to library books' (Sydney Morning Herald 1900h, 8).

The fumigation of coastal vessels to try to kill imported rats began on the initiative of private shipping companies as rumours circulated of plague's global spread. By March 16th a dedicated team was assembled under Superintendent of Fumigation Mr N. Lockyer to undertake mandatory fumigation for all ships arriving in Australia or travelling from Sydney to other ports in Australia, for which they needed a 'fumigation certificate' (Ashburton-Thompson 1900b, 15–16). Notwithstanding the futility of the method, on April 3rd the Board of Water Supply and Sewerage began fumigating the sewers (see Figure 8). While Ashburton-Thompson praised the adequacy of the

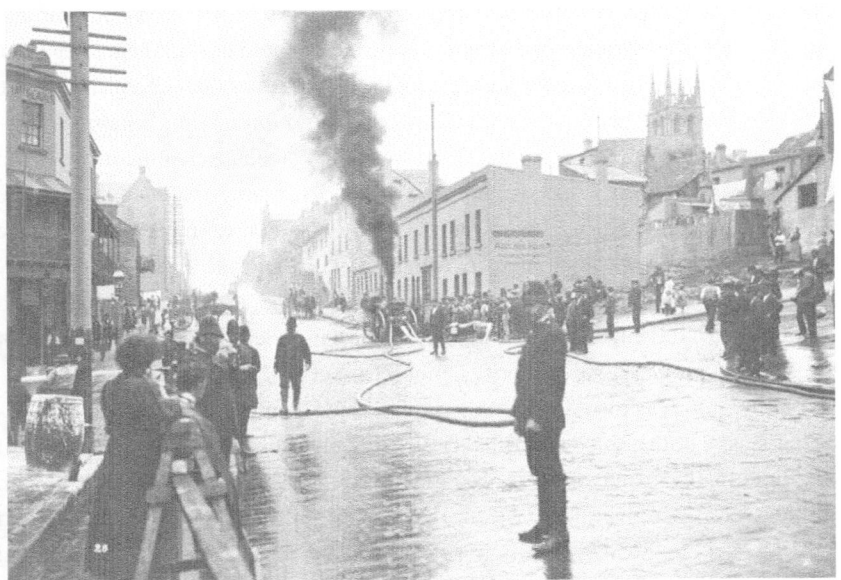

Figure 8 Views taken during Cleansing Operations, Kent Street, Sydney, 1900,
Vol. I. Under the supervision of Mr George McCredie, NSW. 1900. Image
courtesy: Collections of the State Library of New South Wales.

suburban sewerage network, he claimed that by contrast between 20,000 and
21,000 of the 22,000 sewerage connections in the city were 'improper, imper-
fect and dangerous', discharging directly onto the harbour foreshores
(Ashburton-Thompson 1900b, 46). While the thousands of sewers were
blown with sulphur fumes and flushed with chloride of lime, they produced
only 300 to 400 rat bodies. Yet chemical quantities were so excessive that
Darling Harbour filled with dead fish (Echenberg 2007, 253). The only real
benefit of the process was that the smell of sulphur helped McCreadie's team
identify weak points in the sewerage network. Ashburton-Thompson said, 'an
incidental and useful effect of the fumigation was to fix the position of many
faults in the old system, through which the fumes escaped so as to be strongly
perceived within houses, and even in the open' (Ashburton-Thompson 1900b,
46). He may have just been feeling a spike in morale at the temporary compre-
hensiveness of the method.

  Fumigation technologies were also put to work to rid the city of Buenos Aires
of a comparable plague outbreak (Engelmann et al. 2020, 151). The notable
difference between Sydney and Buenos Aires in the nineteenth century was that
Sydney had a reputation for being dirty, while Buenos Aires was supposed to
have been clean (Engelmann et al. 2020, 159). In Buenos Aires, Marot

Machines were purchased to pump the city full of sulphur. With the discovery of bacteria the objective of these works went from hiding disgusting smells to eradicating pests (Engelmann et al. 2020, 165, 171). The symbolic work of the odour of formalin, sulphur, or chloride was to act on the frightened imaginations of people. Fumigation replaced odours identified as disgusting with those which represented modern purification, allaying the sense of abject fear and disgust which pervaded the city at that time (Engelmann et al. 2020, 164). Over time the project in both Buenos Aires and Sydney moved offshore, as maritime quarantine and fumigation became the focus of disease control and containment measures, as historian Alison Bashford has demonstrated (Bashford 1998; Bashford 2004).

6.4 New Postcolonial Sensory Order of the City

The historiography of smell in nineteenth- and twentieth-century sanitation reform is contested, with the key issue being whether sanitation reform eliminated or changed the odours of the city. Reinarz and Classen et al. have claimed that in nineteenth-century Europe, sanitary crises resulted in urban reform across Europe that created a new standard of 'olfactory neutrality' (Classen et al. 1994, 81; Reinarz 2014, 179). In psychoanalyst Dominique Laporte's history of the privatisation of waste in France, the relegation of waste and certain odours to the private household transformed the threshold of tolerance for certain odours (Laporte 2000, 66). Historian Alain Corbin refers to this process in comparable terms as 'lowering of olfactory tolerance' (Corbin 1986, 59). In *Aroma: The Cultural History of Smell*, Classen et al. substantiate this claim that there was a transformation in the threshold of tolerance to odours with sanitation reform in the late nineteenth century and the changing role of the public sphere in cities. As public space was democratised, they argue, smell regulated social divisions and rendered them socially intelligible. This resulted in people becoming more attuned to organic odour, like the odours of the human body or domesticated animals (see Figure 9), and more likely to note the source of a bad odour (Classen et al. 1994, 81–2). Robert Jütte also claims that cities in Germany became more odourless from 1915 over the course of the twentieth century. Courts interpreted excess as whatever local residents claimed was abnormal, which 'implied a new "sensory" interpretation of "local norms" which remained in force until 1959, when the passage referring to "normal local levels" was amended' (Jütte 2018, 171). These initial signs of deodorisation gave way to 'a process of reodorization', which Jütte argues was characterised by the repression of unpleasant odours and the production of fragrance (Jütte 2018, 185).

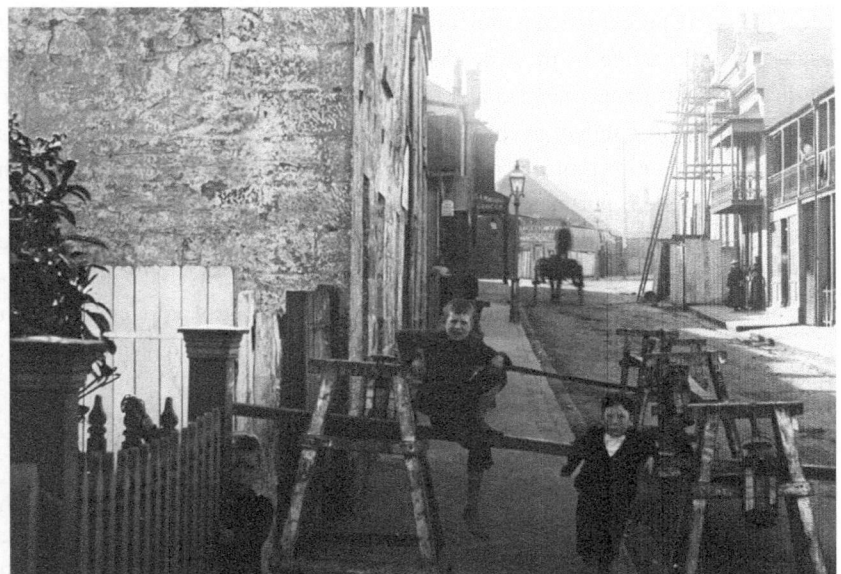

Figure 9 Street scene in Myrtle Street Chippendale [A-00036141]. City of SydneyDemolition Books, 1900. Image courtesy: City of Sydney Archives.

Yet a number of historians have proposed an antithesis, arguing that smell and odours continued to be present and powerful in western cities in the twentieth century or that secular positivism resulted in the decline of smell (Jenner 2011, 335–51). Mark Smith notes Jenner's efforts in successfully destabilising the assumed binary between societies before and after sanitary reform as either odiferous or deodorised (Smith 2018a, xv). Jenner argues 'deodorisation' is a misleading term which confuses the removal of specific odours associated with industry and human waste with the removal of all odours from public space (Jenner 2011, 340–1). He argues that 'to suggest that nineteenth-and twentieth-century sanitary developments amounted to a "total war on smells" on the part of modernity is thoroughly misleading, because the modern (however defined) embraced and emitted so many of them' (Jenner 2011, 340). Boddice and Smith, take a more centrist position, arguing that an inodorous state was preferred in the twentieth century, while the smells of antiseptic and disinfectant were tolerated (Boddice et al. 2020, 42). Melanie Kiechle argues that American cities continued to smell and that these smells yielded power in everyday life long after sanitation reform (Kiechle 2016, 763). Yet there were changes in how the perception of odour was valued. With technological and scientific innovation, people's perceptions of poor air quality and reports of bad odours were invalidated in the courts, which favoured formalist, empirical measurements or expert testimony. Without 'expert corroboration', an individual account of bad odour could become a source of doubt (Kiechle 2016, 765). Bad odours went from being a very local issue, regulated by local courts attributing responsibility to the source of an odour at individual, household, or building level, to being viewed as a regional problem regulated between metropolitan boards of health and industry (Kiechle 2016, 767). Nonetheless, she argues, smell continued to be a common sense that people relied upon to understand which places and people harboured harmful germs (Kiechle 2016, 766). In New York, a sense of miasmatic dread did not evaporate with germ theory; it was reinforced by better understanding of the presence of microbes and how they caused disease.

This Element maintains that during this disease outbreak in Sydney there was a very keen desire for new odours. The city reeked of sulphur, perchloride of mercury, carbolic acid, and chloride of lime while streets, houses, sewers, and wharves were fumigated, scrubbed, and washed down. Lasting change following the outbreak resulted from the process of extending the sewerage network to inner city premises. The Sydney Harbour Trust was established to take statutory responsibility for all the private wharves around the city harbours and oversee their reconstruction, which was recommended by Ashburton-Thompson (Ashburton-Thompson 1900b). At the same time, the Darling Harbour Wharves Resumption Act was passed in late 1900, to facilitate the demolition and reconstruction of properties (see Figure 10) around

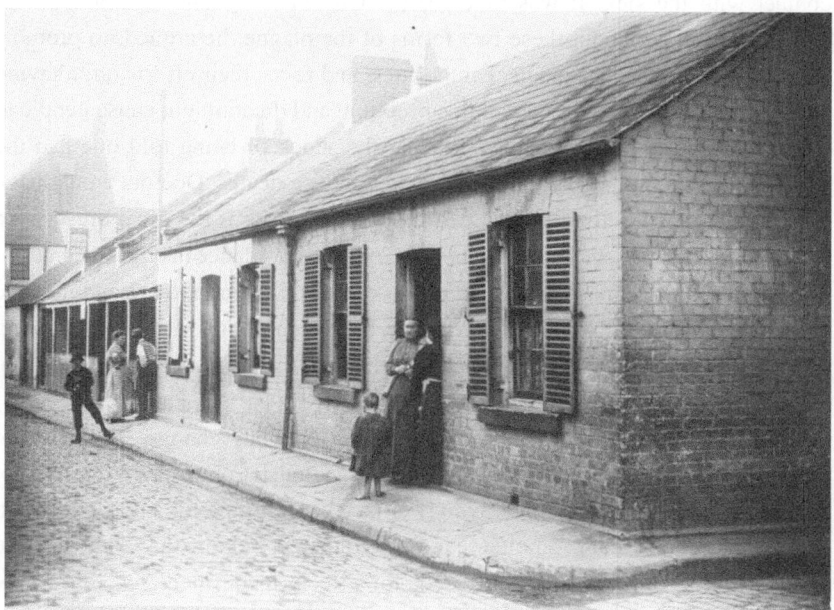

Figure 10 Resumed houses 2–10 Athlone Place Ultimo [A-00036122]. City of Sydney Demolition Books, 1900. Image courtesy: City of Sydney Archives.

the harbourside wharves (NSW Government 1900). Legislation around noxious trades was slowly strengthened, gradually pushing these industries further out of the centre and into areas which were exclusively zoned for industrial use rather than a mix of industrial and residential uses. Ongoing demand for public works, and replacement of horses with motor cars, meant that post-plague Sydney smelt of tarred metal, asphalt, and other materials used to repair roads and footpaths, rather than the horse manures and stables more common in the nineteenth century. Fumigation became increasingly common in domestic or commercial spaces such as boarding houses. By late 1901 new complaints had begun to surface about the city's 'smoke nuisance', describing the high volume of smoke that arose from chimneys and funnels both from houses on land and ships on the harbour (Sydney Morning Herald 1901, 7). Rather than removing smells or deodorising the city, demand to transform the odours identified with disease resulted in a new urban landscape of odours and new concerns.

7 Mediating Affect

On the 6th of May 1900, a concerned citizen wrote a letter to the *Sydney Morning Herald*. He claimed that two forms of the plague existed: a pulmonary form, which could be transmitted by breath, such as the form found in India; and another form currently circulating around Sydney, which was not communicated by contact with the sick. It was time for the Citizen's Vigilance Committees to educate the public about these two forms of the plague, he argued, to promote the views of the leading medical authorities, and focus their efforts on 'allaying panic'. Indeed, he thought that all this brooding and dread might cause people to imagine they are afflicted, or, worse, that the shock of being told one had the plague could precipitate symptoms and even induce death. 'Doctors would have a better chance of pulling the patient through the attack if the great dread were removed and the patient's spirits kept up'. Fear and avoidance had far too great an impact on the city: 'many ladies are positively afraid to go to town, and in some cases I know of hardly care to go outside their own door for fear of knocking against someone who had the plague and thus contracting it' (Sydney Morning Herald 1900i, 6).

Emotions produce and are products of history. They change. They do not proceed in a linear direction, between cultures, countries or times (Frevert 2016, 62). In his letter, this concerned Sydney citizen was arguing for a new education campaign, not one that promoted fear and avoidance, but one that allayed it. He advocated for emotion to be diffused, for affects to be mediated, by a new awareness and education regarding the certainty of the threat. Emotion remained politically important and useful, however, throughout the event.

This Element has examined how emotions and affects can be strategically evoked and deployed to justify interventions and compel behaviour change. I wish to highlight the plasticity of the disgust response to show how the combination of context, meaning, and judgement combine to inform what it is we call disgusting and judge worthy of intervention. These emotions and the responses they demand are therefore not *a priori* given, waiting to be unveiled, but actively generated and produced by the discursive, material and embodied context as the crisis gives way to a contestation over power. Emotions can change as a result of and even during an outbreak of disease due to their plasticity. As Boddice and Smith argue, 'emotions are not politically stable in light of disease, and it is the specificity of context that allows us to see and detect shifts' (Boddice et al. 2020, 42). A transforming context actively intervenes in and changes sensitivities and the ways in which people respond to things, educating feelings, for better or worse.

Uncertainty in the provenance, ecology, treatment or prevention of contagious and non-contagious diseases can compel the use of the emotional and affective power of symbolism to authorise hypotheses and conjecture. Fluctuating concepts of what constitutes dirt solicits an affective reaction which embodies these categories, making them seem natural or inevitable, and requiring a form of sublimation or aversion in response. In the first outbreak of the plague in Sydney, this was to the clear detriment of marginalised people, including Chinese immigrants and the urban poor, animals like the rat, odours and locations across the city that became disgust objects.

7.1 Disgust, Toxicity and Medical Materialism

One of the reasons why this symbol of dirt and the variable category of secondary disgust objects are so powerful is because they can be traced back to or associated with primary or core disgust objects, which in some cases can cause us harm. On Sunday 8th April in the *Sunday Times*, a few months after plague was first detected in Sydney, an editorial warned readers to pay more attention to the state of the jugs in which they serve milk, which left unattended on doorsteps and window ledges, 'gather germs of typhoid or tuberculosis, which fly about with the dust' (Sunday Times 1900b, 1). While the scientific understanding of contamination is weak, there is a possibility that spoiled milk would contain microbes that make a person sick.

It is this kind of observation that has given rise to various theses and antitheses regarding the idea that the disgust reaction evolved to support pathogen avoidance (Rozin et al. 2016, 818). On the one hand, Panksepp argues that disgust is a universal affective process, not only in humans, but in all mammals, which help them 'sense conditions that need to be avoided in order to prevent disease'

(Panksepp 2007, 1826). He claims that disgust is more akin to a sensory affect – like hunger, thirst, nausea, fatigue and many other bodily states or 'tools of the nervous system' – than a culturally specific emotion (Panksepp 2007, 1819). Yet this Element concurs with Rozin et al. that core disgust did not evolve as a result of pathogen avoidance because disgust is a learned reaction, which is why it cannot be equated with other drives like hunger, nausea and thirst (Rozin et al. 2016, 819). They argue that cooking food, purifying water and antibiotic drugs are all pathogen avoidance behaviours that are explicitly cultural and subject to change with new information (Rozin et al. 2016, 819). Likewise Tybur et al. claim that disgust is not based upon pathogen avoidance as there are many activities humans undertake which can easily transmit bacteria or infections but do not elicit a disgust response (Tybur et al. 2020, 12).

Rottman et al. also argue that pathogen avoidance is an insufficient theory to explain the origins of the disgust response, as not only do people often fail to be disgusted by objects that could cause disease, but 'the line between dangerous pathogen and helpful bacteria can be murky' (Rottman et al. 2020, 29). New research which examines a cultural shift from antibiotic to probiotic notions of self and culture indicates that avoiding pathogens may even be detrimental (Greenhough et al. 2018, 1). Greenhough et al. argue that by contrast with the antibiotic, antimicrobial world view promoted by sanitation reform, hygiene and public and health, 'probiotic cultures (in the sense of particular human-non human collectives) can be enduring, reflecting long histories of human-microbe collaboration' (Greenhough et al. 2018, 2). Instead, I maintain that disgust as affect or emotion is a means to preserve and produce identity by distancing us from any reminders of the certainty that we will die (Rozin et al. 2016, 819). While the odour of decay or death may be some of the most potent disgust triggers, any aversion to them are more likely a reaction to existential threats, as Kristeva would maintain, psychic terror or threats to identity rather than the likely presence of pathogenic bacteria (Rozin et al. 2016, 819). That is not to say that hygienic and defensive acts have no place. Disgust and its consequential hygienic acts do protect us from harmful germs, but protection from all germs would result in dysbiosis, an imbalance between human-microbial relations. Disgust must be endlessly flexible, recalibrated, or rebalanced to allow for our ongoing shared existence with microbes (Greenhough et al. 2018, 2). We must learn to sense both the risks and rewards of living with microbes (Greenhough et al. 2018, 5). On a personal level, after a strong reaction to using antibiotics against *Yersinia enterocolitica*, my doctor, my gastroenterologist and I all agreed to attempt to manage a secondary infection of Aeromonas which I came down with a month later using probiotics and aiming for a reduction in stress. Wiping things off or casting them out can cause new problems.

As the case study of the Sydney plague demonstrates, the range of situations and circumstances which can provoke disgust are much wider than mere pathogen avoidance and – importantly – the expression of disgust is not always triggered by pathogenic objects. Rather it is informed by whatever a given culture and time consider symbolic of anomaly or disorder and therefore threatening to identity (Kristeva 1982, 10). Rozin et al. consider this question in their discussion of whether disgust originated as a response to noxious food and was gradually associated with more contexts, situations and objects (Rozin et al. 1987, 22; Rozin et al. 2016, 815; Tomkins 1962, 128). Yet harmless or even nutritious item of food might be disgusting simply because of its history or the context, who has handled it or where and how it is served. These practices may result in food being regarded as contaminated, even though it could well be beneficial. Disgust is not strictly applied to food, or things that are tasted or ingested, or things that are noxious. Disgust is a response to anything that threatens identity. Likewise Douglas rejects the argument that the repulsion by dirt is mere 'pathogen avoidance', claiming it is unnecessarily reductive and insufficient to account for all the aesthetic and spiritual explanations of hygienic rules (Douglas 1966, 29). While she admits that sometimes rituals are symbolic and hygienic, she thinks that there is always a concurrent interpretation of ritual or symbolic acts (Douglas 1966, 32). 'Even if some of Moses's dietary rules were hygienically beneficial', she says, 'it is a pity to treat him as an enlightened public health administrator, rather than as a spiritual leader' (Douglas 1966, 29). The ritual rules which may be defined as 'medical materialism' express beliefs which guard against dangers that go beyond verifiable harm to the body, which is to say, the dangers of a disordered world (Douglas 1966, 32). In 1900 Sydney, as in other instances of uncertainty, medical science did not know exactly what the threat was and was not always able to convince the public of its best guesses. In this instance, there was less coincidence between material threat and sym-bolic meaning, so the sense of threat was mapped onto the marginalised, disempowered, or anything anomalous to the desired order.

7.2 Disgust and Agency

This Element makes the case that there is a need to understand and draw attention to the question of how temporality informs our apparently urgent physiological, affective, and emotional responses as we learn and unlearn new information during infectious disease outbreaks. The way disgust was instru-mentalised in the 1900 Sydney plague is evidence of its plasticity. Affects may be tricky to change but it is possible, nothing is inevitable (Reddy 1997, 330). Solomon's view that emotions are a rational response to an unusual situation would reinforce the view that we can learn and modify our affective responses. Indeed, Solomon would argue that there is no primary disgust object, that all of our emotional responses can be mediated by the work of individual reason and will (Solomon 2003, 11). This is a very strong view. The role of judgement in influencing the disgust process would give us some agency in how we respond to things emotionally, though this agency is mediated by the strong weight of habit and other factors that distinguish our bodies biologically, historically, and culturally. As Carel argues, many everyday routine actions are pre-reflexive – the product of habit rather than conscious reflection (Carel 2016, 22). We do not have pure agency, but there may be a fit between an emotion and a person's history, culture, character, or, as Solomon himself says, 'it is a conception of freedom and responsibility that makes sense in terms of the narrative of one's life' (Solomon 2003, 204). An emotion that fits into this culturally situated narrative is one that we are responsible for, even if it is spontaneous.

I have claimed that the learnings and evaluations which inform the disgust reaction happen at a different time to the reaction itself. A more conscious evaluation of an object as disgusting produces an emotional response. An affective or immediate response is spontaneous, but still informed by the discourse, language, and knowledge that people engage with on a day-to-day basis, as well as their experiences and habits. The granular work of analysing disgust teaches us that an affect can be both involuntary and learned, or the product of judgement. It is just that these two activities, the judgement and the reaction, occur at different times, they are not simultaneous. We can read about something one day and then have a disgust reaction to it a week later without remembering or realising what the original influence was – that is to say, the source of our education in disgust. Our everyday values, assessments, and judgements will inform what we find disgusting in an encounter. Yet new priorities and information can overcome disgust, including a desire for connection with others. These evaluations were evident in Sydney on many occasions, in the decision to release the hospital staff from quarantine because they were essential workers, in the refusal to kiss a Bible recently handled by someone released from quarantine, in the temporary preference for doing business by telephone rather than in person. Yet the duality of disgust and desire may result in the dissolution of the self into the other with other affects, such as love. Rozin and Fallon are among those who argue that bodily substances that would be considered disgusting among strangers could be neutral or a source of pleasure between parents and their children, or between lovers. They claim, '[i]n the case of both lovers and children, the source of the object can be considered an extension of the biological self' (Rozin et al. 1987, 26–7). With the dissolution of identity into the other there is no frantic effort to maintain boundaries through separation from or from another's bodily substances. Disgust and distance are overcome by love (Rozin et al. 1987, 26; Rozin et al. 2016, 828).

7.3 Intentional Disgust

As identified in the introduction to this Element, an investigation into the plasticity of disgust can shed some valuable light on the other debates within history of emotions that have become almost intractable. To begin with, one of Ruth Leys' criticisms of what she considers the unwarranted popularity of the term affect is that it implies that affect is not intentional (Leys 2011, 437–8). There is a question of moral responsibility and will if emotions are involuntary or unintentional responses to other things and beings. My claim regarding the changing dynamics and ontologies of disgust is an answer to her claim. Even if disgust is experienced as involuntary in a specific moment, we can still be intentional about how we evaluate the world to challenge and change our understandings of what is disgusting. These responses are influenced by how we think about and symbolise objects around us and depend on culture, history, and experience.

The benefit of moving beyond strict understandings of concepts as either intentional or unintentional is that it restores a certain kind of agency to the environment around us (Irwin 2010, 36; Plumwood 2009, 117; Rees 2017, 2). One of the reasons the concept of affect appealed to so many theorists was that it was a way of overcoming the limits of subjectivity, which cut us off from others, rejecting kinship, the intersubjective, shared ground (Brennan 2004, 119). As Pedwell argues, 'for many critical thinkers, affect is precisely that which radically exceeds 'the human' – and therefore it may not make sense to assess such theories using psychological terms referring to human-centred terms and processes' (Pedwell 2020, 139). If we acknowledge the agency of the world around us, of the affects that influence us, we release ourselves from the isolating notion that a person and their emotions are completely self-contained and self-generated (Rees 2017, 3). As Brennan writes so eloquently, 'affects are in the air as well as the individual psyche. We carry them in the earliest recesses of memory, but we also encounter them in the street. These affects are what threaten the discreteness of the persons, the things that divert their psyches (or souls) from their distinct paths and ways of being' (Brennan 2004, 113). It gives us an important way out, and a pathway to forgiveness for those moments of affective failure or transgression (Brennan 2004, 95).

Of the ten outbreaks of the plague that occurred in Sydney between 1900 and 1921, only the first outbreak was managed as though it were contagious. By the 1901 outbreak, Ashburton-Thompson already had an opportunity to analyse data from 1900 and to conclude with confidence that it was not contagious. 'It has been shown that the epidemic of 1900 was not caused by direct communication with the sick, nor by diffusion of infected articles, nor by place infection. These observations on the mode of spread we have now had opportunity of checking. They have been confirmed and amplified' (New South Wales Board of Health et al. 1902, 1). As a result, in the subsequent two epidemics in 1901 and 1902 Ashburton-Thompson ceased to segregate contacts of the sick, instead defining a 'contact' as someone who had been in close proximity with plague rats. The changing definition led to a focus on disinfection of clothing and housing. Ashburton-Thompson was adamant that a corollary of this changing policy was 'a great saving of time, anxiety, perturbation of the public mind . . . the business of managing the second epidemic proceeded quietly and steadily, without excitement on the one hand and without opposition to necessary measures on the other' (Ashburton-Thompson 1903, 1090). The authority of and confidence in the institution of public health had been resolutely established.

The year 1900 was a formative time in Sydney, the end of the century, and the final year before the self-governing colonies were federated in the Commonwealth of Australia. In Sydney, the governance enacted through the institution of public health succeeded in protecting people from the plague by limiting transmission within the city and dramatically transforming the physical and sensory landscape. For the first time, the Board of Health exercised its new powers under the Public Health Act to ward off the threat of disease and the public crisis it provoked. The successful response established its authority within New South Wales and Australia more broadly. Public health came to intervene in affairs of state from the management of borders, immigration, and national identity through quarantine, to the management and regulation of streets, waterfronts, homes, and individuals as they circulated through the city.

When the six British colonies became one nation on 1st January 1901, the only public health power granted to the new Commonwealth government in the constitution regarded quarantine. All other powers were retained by the state governments and their Boards of Health (Bashford 1998, 388). As Bashford has established, this public health thinking also deeply informed the formation of the nation. Australia was characterised as clean and hygienic 'in which island stood for immunity', in opposition to polluted or diseased geographical neighbours, that is to say, 'a pure national self, and a pathologized, contaminated and racialised other' (Bashford 1998, 397). Fear of immigration was explicitly framed as a fear of disease. One of the first Acts passed by the new federal government was the 1901 Immigration Restriction Act, which not only placed almost impossible restrictions on the immigration of non-British immigrants, but explicitly prohibited entry to Australia of 'any person suffering from an infectious or contagious disease of a loathsome or dangerous character' (Bashford 1998, 398).

This had a profound impact on the identity of the colony of New South Wales as it transformed into the Federation of Australia, providing public health with considerable authority and basing citizenship in the new nation on ideas of behaviour and health which were tied up with assumptions about race. In this historical moment, the prevalence of the symbolism of dirt and filth became a platform for change, to produce a social order suitable for a new nation distinct from other colonies of the British Empire, and a social identity suitable for its citizens.

This is not an exhaustive study but rather exploratory, partial, and somewhat creative in both its analysis and conclusion. One interesting direction for further research would be to explore the question of resistance to this power. How did the local Chinese populations respond to these acts of subjugation explored in Section 3? Hitzer identifies the problem with understanding the experiences of the so-called human objects of disgust, such as cancer patients, because the vulnerable and socially marginalised were not considered subjects with a point of view that should be documented and recorded. She argues, 'it may have simply seemed inconceivable that people who were seen by society as repulsive or disgusting could themselves feel disgust' (Hitzer 2020, 160). What forms of psychic defences or forms of resistance were palpable and active during the first outbreak of the plague in Sydney as so many people lost their homes? As much as possible I have tried to describe the cynicism and heterogeneity of opinion among Sydney's residents, yet there are other possibile ways of researching their inevitably diverse takes on this experience.

I have regrettably had little opportunity to explore questions of how disgust and desire operate together. Questions of consumption and hunger could also emerge from a study of disgust. How does the inverse of this emotion attempt to produce intimacy or identification with those of desired objects and places? I have clearly been limited to how disgust was mobilised by the use of symbolism in English language texts. Another direction for research could be to consider different subjectivities or non-verbal experiences of disgust. And another research question would perhaps consider how humans can learn to positively, rather than negatively, sense or notice the presence of microbes or toxins. Finally, ongoing attention to how emotions and affects are deliberately solicited in public health communication would be helpful to understand both the value of these approaches and their risks. With the institution of public health and the authority of medicine yielding considerable cultural power, it is very important to be alive to what happens when the knowledge informing that power is shifting or changing.

If the Covid-19 pandemic has shown us anything it is that medical practitioners and people with institutional authority do not always have knowledge about a disease or how it is caused, prevented, and treated in the early stages of a pandemic. They are flying blind, they are uncertain, and the decisions they make are informed by emotions, assumptions, and symbols. I noticed the parallels in some of the emotional patterns of the Covid-19 pandemic, particularly the panic in the early response, and later in the disgust people began to feel at not only social, but physiological, interactions with other people. I wondered what work these adverse reactions were doing to the social or body politics in which they were playing out. I lived through this event in Sydney, and I could see the repression of specific groups or identity depending on geography, race, risk, tolerance once again. What happens when we no longer trust shared spaces, when we do not want to risk an interaction or an exchange, when we experience fear, disgust, and aversion to the presence of others? This project reflects on some of these questions, with reference to the specificities of the plague in Sydney in 1900 but with some indicators or ways of thinking about our own experiences too.

References

Anderson, W. 1995. Excremental Colonialism: Public Health and the Poetics of Pollution. *Critical Inquiry* 21(3): 640–69.

Anon. 1907. Plague and Fleas. *Nature* 77(1986): 59–60.

Arnold, D. 1982. *Touching the Body: Perspectives on Plague*. R. Guha (ed.). Delhi: Oxford University Press.

Ashburton-Thompson, J. 1900a. An Account of the Epidemic of Plague at Sydney. *Public Health* 13: 1–20.

Ashburton-Thompson, J. 1900b. *Map of Portion of Sydney and Suburbs Showing by Coloured Spots the Probable Place of Infection in 225 Cases of Plague* [Cartographic Material]. Sydney: Dept. of Lands.

Ashburton-Thompson, J. 1900c. Report on an Outbreak of the Plague in Sydney New South Wales. In *Votes and Proceedings of the Legislative Assembly*, 7–80. New South Wales Government Printer.

Ashburton-Thompson, J. 1901. A Contribution to the Aetiology of Plague. *The Journal of Hygiene* 1(2): 153–67. www.jstor.org/stable/4618399 [Accessed 8 October 2021].

Ashburton-Thompson, J. 1903. On the Eitology of Bubonic Plague: An Epidemiological Contribution. *The Lancet* 162(4181): 1090–2.

Ashburton-Thompson, J. 1904. Plague at Sydney: To the Editor of Public Health. *Public Health* XVI(9): 45.

Ashburton-Thompson, J. 1906. On the Epidemiology of Plague. *The Journal of Hygiene* 6(5): 537–69.

Ashburton-Thompson, J. 1907a. Protection of India from Invasion by Plague. *BMJ* 2(2451): 1770–1.

Ashburton-Thompson, J. 1907b. The Mode of Spread and the Prevention of Plague in Australia. *The Lancet* 170(4390): 1104–7.

Ashmead, A. 1901. Original Communications: Synopsis of Dr. J. Ashburton Thompson's Report of Plague in New South Wales. *Missouri Medical and Surgical Journal* LXXXI(1): 9–14.

Australian Star. 1900a. Citizen's Vigilance Committee. *Australian Star*. http://nla.gov.au/nla.news-article229381266 [Accessed 22 October 2021].

Australian Star. 1900b. The Council and the Plague. *Australian Star*. http://nla.gov.au/nla.news-article229381267 [Accessed 22 October 2021].

Baker, G. 1900. *Inspector of Nuisances – Town Clerk: Annual Report for 1899*. https://archives.cityofsydney.nsw.gov.au/nodes/view/766854 [Accessed 14 December 2021].

Bashford, A. 1998. Quarantine and the Imagining of the Australian Nation. *Health* 2(4): 387–402.

Bashford, A. 2004. *Imperial Hygiene a Critical History of Colonialism, Nationalism and Public Health*. Houndsmills: Palgrave Macmillan.

Bashford, A., & Strange, C. 2007. Thinking Historically about Public Health. *Medical Humanities* 33(2): 87–92.

Boddice, R., & Hitzer, B. 2022. Emotion and Experience in the History of Medicine: Elaborating a Theory and Seeking a Method. In R. Boddice & B. Hitzer (eds.), *Feeling Dis-Ease in Modern History: Experiencing Medicine and Illness*, 3–19. History of Emotions, London: Bloomsbury.

Boddice, R., & Smith, M. M. 2020. *Emotion, Sense, Experience*. Cambridge: Cambridge University Press.

Borthwick, F. 2000. Olfaction and Taste: Invasive Odours and Disappearing Objects. *The Australian Journal of Anthropology* 11(2): 127–40.

Bourdieu, P. 1977. *Outline of a Theory of Practice*. Cambridge: Cambridge University Press.

Brennan, T. 2004. *The Transmission of Affect*. Ithaca: Cornell University Press.

Carel, H. 2016. *Phenomenology of Illness*. 1st ed. Oxford: Oxford University Press.

Classen, C., Howes, D., & Synnott, A. 1994. *Aroma: The Cultural History of Smell*. Abingdon: Routledge.

Collins, F. M. 1996. Pasteurella, Yersinia, and Francisella. In S. Baron (ed.), *Medical Microbiology*, Galveston: University of Texas Medical Branch at Galveston. www.ncbi.nlm.nih.gov/books/NBK7798/ [Accessed 23 September 2022].

Corbin, A. 1986. *The Foul and the Fragrant Odor and the French Social Imagination*. Cambridge, MA: Harvard University Press.

Cumberland Argus. 1900. Infection and the Railways. *Cumberland Argus and Fruitgrowers Advocate*. http://nla.gov.au/nla.news-article85822028 [Accessed 25 November 2021].

Cummins, C. J. 2003. *A History of Medical Administration in NSW 1788 – 1973*. North Sydney: NSW Department of Health. www.health.nsw.gov.au/about/history/Publications/history-medical-admin.pdf.

Curson, P. 1985. *Times of Crisis: Epidemics in Sydney 1788–1900*. Sydney: Sydney University Press.

Curson, P., & McCracken, K. W. J. 1989. *Plague in Sydney: The Anatomy of an Epidemic*. Kensington: New South Wales University Press.

Curtis, V. A. 2007. Dirt, Disgust and Disease: A Natural History of Hygiene. *Journal of Epidemiology & Community Health* 61(8): 660–4. https://jech-bmj-com.simsrad.net.ocs.mq.edu.au/content/61/8/660 [Accessed 13 April 2023].

Daily Telegraph. 1900. The City Council Startled. *Daily Telegraph*, 7. http://nla.gov.au/nla.news-article237173353 [Accessed 30 January 2023].

Dixon, T. 2003. *From Passions to Emotions: The Creation of a Secular Psychological Category*. Cambridge: Cambridge University Press.

Douglas, M. 1966. *Purity and Danger: An Analysis of Concepts of Pollution and Taboo*. London: Routledge & Kegan Paul.

Echenberg, M. 2002. Pestis Redux: The Initial Years of the Third Bubonic Plague Pandemic, 1894–1901. *Journal of World History* 13(2): 429–50. https://go-gale-com.ezproxy.sl.nsw.gov.au/ps/i.do?p=AONE&sw=w&issn=10456007&v=2.1&it=r&id=GALE%7CA91271526&sid=googleScholar&linkaccess=abs [Accessed 8 October 2021].

Echenberg, M. 2007. *Plague Ports: The Global Urban Impact of Bubonic Plague, 1894–1901*. New York: New York University Press.

Engelmann, L., & Lynteris, C. 2020. *Sulphuric Utopias: A History of Maritime Fumigation*. Cambridge, MA: The MIT Press.

Enzensberger, C. 1972. *Smut: An Anatomy of Dirt*. London: Calder and Boyars.

Evening News. 1900a. Parramatta's Sanitary Condition. *Evening News*. http://nla.gov.au/nla.news-article117031404 [Accessed 22 October 2021].

Evening News. 1900b. The Plague. *Evening News*. http://nla.gov.au/nla.news-article117031347 [Accessed 22 October 2021].

Evening News. 1900c. Those Filthy Bank Notes. *Evening News*. http://nla.gov.au/nla.news-article113710908 [Accessed 29 October 2021].

Evening News. 1900d. The Plague, Mid Winter Sale, The Mutual Stores, Pitt Street. *Evening News*, 8. http://nla.gov.au/nla.news-article113716705 [Accessed 29 January 2023].

Fitzgerald, S. 1987. *Rising Damp: Sydney 1870–90*. Melbourne: Oxford University Press.

Fletcher, W. H. 1900. Manly M.C. Forwarding Copy of Letter Sent to Board of Health re Refuse Coming Ashore. https://archives.cityofsydney.nsw.gov.au/nodes/view/770935 [Accessed 14 December 2021].

Foucault, M. 1975. *The Birth of the Clinic an Archaeology of Medical Perception*. New York: Vintage Books.

Foucault, M. 1977. *Discipline and Punish: The Birth of the Prison*. London: Allen Lane.

Frevert, U. 2016. The History of Emotions. In L. F. Barrett, M. Lewis, & J. M. Haviland-Jones (eds.), *Handbook of Emotions, Fourth Edition*, 49–65. New York: Guilford. http://ebookcentral.proquest.com/lib/mqu/detail.action?docID=4406910 [Accessed 14 June 2022].

Fuchs, T. 2013. Existential Vulnerability: Toward a Psychopathology of Limit Situations. *Psychopathology* 46(5): 301–8. www.proquest.com/docview/1464752916/abstract/8C60FDB8A2A84D70PQ/1 [Accessed 29 January 2023].

Gell, A. 1975. *Metamorphosis of the Cassowaries: Umeda Society, Language and Ritual.* London: Athlone Press.

Greenhough, B., Dwyer, A., Grenyer, R. Hodgetts, T., McLeod, C., & Lorimer, J. 2018. Unsettling Antibiosis: How Might Interdisciplinary Researchers Generate a Feeling for the Microbiome and to What Effect? *Palgrave Communications* 4(1): 1–12. www.nature.com/articles/s41599-018-0196-3 [Accessed 25 January 2023].

Hirst, J. B. 1988. *The Strange Birth of Colonial Democracy: New South Wales 1848–1884.* Sydney: Allen & Unwin.

Hitzer, B. 2020. The Odor of Disgust: Contemplating the Dark Side of 20th-Century Cancer History. *Emotion Review* 12(3): 156–67.

Hitzer, B. 2022. History Before Corona: Memory, Experience and Emotions. In R. Boddice & B. Hitzer (eds.), *Feeling Dis-Ease in Modern History: Experiencing Medicine and Illness*, 61–84. History of Emotions, London: Bloomsbury.

Irwin, R. 2010. *Climate Change and Philosophy: Transformational Possibilities.* London: Bloomsbury.

Isen, A. M., & Diamond, G. A. 1989. Affect and Automaticity. In J. S. Uleman & J. A. Bargh (eds.), *Unintended Thought*, 124–152. New York: The Guilford Press

Jenner, M. S. R. 2011. Follow Your Nose? Smell, Smelling, and Their Histories. *The American Historical Review* 116(2): 335–51. https://doi.org/10.1086/ahr.116.2.335 [Accessed 21 November 2021].

Jones, M. O. 2000. What's Disgusting, Why, and What Does It Matter? *Journal of Folklore Research* 37(1): 53–71.

Jütte, R. 2018. Reodorizing the Modern Age. In M. M. Smith (ed.), *Smell and History: A Reader*, 170–186. Morgantown: West Virginia University Press.

Kaster, B. 2001. The Dynamics of Fastidium and the Ideology of Disgust. *Transactions of the American Philological Association* 113: 143–189.

Kelly, M. 1981. *Plague Sydney 1900: A Photographic Introduction to a Hidden Sydney, 1900.* Sydney: Doak Press.

Kiechle, M. 2016. Navigating by Nose: Fresh Air, Stench Nuisance, and the Urban Environment, 1840–1880. *Journal of Urban History* 42(4): 753–71.

Kirmayer, L. J. 1993. Healing and the Invention of Metaphor: The Effectiveness of Symbols Revisited. *Culture, Medicine and Psychiatry* 17(2): 161–95.

Kristeva, J. 1982. *Powers of Horror: An Essay on Abjection.* New York: Columbia University Press.

Laporte, D.-G. 2000. *History of Shit.* Cambridge, MA: MIT Press.

Lévi-Strauss, C. 1963. *Structural Anthropology.* New York: Basic Books.

Lewis, I. M. 1977. *Symbols and Sentiments: Cross-Cultural Studies in Symbolism*. London: Academic Press.

Leys, R. 2011. The Turn to Affect: A Critique. *Critical Inquiry* 37(3): 434–72. www.jstor.org/stable/10.1086/659353 [Accessed 30 January 2023].

Leys, R. 2017. *The Ascent of Affect: Genealogy and Critique*. Chicago: University of Chicago Press. www.degruyter.com/document/doi/10.7208/9780226488738/html [Accessed 10 August 2022].

Low, R. B. 1902. *Reports and Papers on Bubonic Plague, by R. Bruce Low: With an Introduction by the Medical Officer of the Local Government Board. An Account of the Progress and Diffusion of Plague Throughout the World, 1898–1901, and of the Measures Employed in Different Countries for Repression of this Disease*. London: H.M. Stationery Office.

Manderson, D. 1997. Substances as Symbols: Race Rhetoric and the Tropes of Australian Drug History. *Social & Legal Studies* 6(3): 383–400.

Massumi, B. 2002. *Parables for the Virtual Movement, Affect, Sensation*. Durham, NC: Duke University Press.

Mauss, M. 1973. Techniques of the Body. *Economy and Society* 2(1): 70–88.

Mayne, A. J. C. 1993. *The Imagined Slum: Newspaper Representation in Three Cities, 1870–1914*. Leicester: Leicester University Press.

Miller, W. I. 1997. *The Anatomy of Disgust*. Cambridge, MA: Harvard University Press.

New South Wales ed. 1883. *Report of the Royal Commission, appointed on the 20th November, 1882, to Inquire into the Nature and Operations of, and to Classify Noxious and Offensive Trades, Within the City of Sydney and its Suburbs, and to Report Generally on Such Trades, Together with the Minutes of Evidence and Appendices*. Sydney: Government Printer.

New South Wales Board of Health, & Ashburton-Thompson, J. 1902. *Report of the Board of Health on a Second Outbreak of Plague at Sydney, 1902*. Sydney: Government Printer.

New South Wales Parliament. 1860. *Condition of the Working Classes of the Metropolis, report from the Select Committee on the Condition of the Working Classes of the Metropolis: together with the Proceedings of the Committee, Minutes of Evidence and Appendix*. Sydney: Thomas Richards, Government Printer.

New South Wales Parliament. 1900a. *Parliamentary Debates / Legislative Council and Legislative Assembly*. Sydney: Government Printer. www.sl.nsw.gov.au/research-and-collections-how-guides/how-use-special-collections [Accessed 1 December 2021].

New South Wales Parliament. 1900b. *Parliamentary Debates / Legislative Council and Legislative Assembly*. Sydney: Government Printer.

www.sl.nsw.gov.au/research-and-collections-how-guides/how-use-spe cial-collections [Accessed 1 December 2021].

NSW Government. 1900. *Darling Harbour Wharves Resumption Act 1900 No 10 – NSW Legislation.* https://legislation.nsw.gov.au/view/whole/html/ repealed/current/act-1900-010 [Accessed 30 January 2023].

Panksepp, J. 2007. Criteria for Basic Emotions: Is Disgust a Primary 'Emotion'? *Cognition & Emotion* 21(8): 1819–28. www.tandfonline.com/ doi/abs/10.1080/02699930701334302 [Accessed 14 June 2022].

Pedwell, C. 2020. Affect Theory's Alternative Genealogies – Review Symposium on Leys's The Ascent of Affect. *History of the Human Sciences* 33(2): 134–42.

Plumwood, V. 2009. Nature in the Active Voice. *Australian Humanities Review* (46): 111–27.

Reddy, W. M. 1997. Against Constructionism: The Historical Ethnography of Emotions. *Current Anthropology* 38(3): 327–51.

Rees, A. 2017. Animal Agents? Historiography, Theory and the History of Science in the Anthropocene. *British Journal for the History of Science Themes* 2: 1–10.

Reinarz, J. 2014. *Past Scents: Historical Perspectives on Smell.* Chicago: University of Illinois Press.

Risse, G. B. 2015. *Driven by Fear: Epidemics and Isolation in San Francisco's House of Pestilence.* Champaign: University of Illinois Press.

Rottman, J., DeJesus, J. M., & Gerdin, E. 2020. The Social Origins of Disgust. In N. Strohminger & V. Kumar (eds.), *The Moral Psychology of Disgust*, London: Rowman & Littlefield International.

Rozin, P., & Fallon, A. E. 1987. A Perspective on Disgust. *Psychological Review* 94(1): 23–41.

Rozin, P., Haidt, J., & McCauley, C. 2016. Disgust. In L. F. Barrett, M. Lewis, & J. M. Haviland-Jones (eds.), *Handbook of Emotions, Fourth Edition*, 815–34. New York: Guilford. http://ebookcentral.proquest.com/lib/mqu/detail .action?docID=4406910 [Accessed 14 June 2022].

Savin, C., Criscuolo, A., Guglielmini, J., Le Guern, A., Carniel, E., Pizarro-Cerda, J., & Brisse, S. 2019. Genus-wide Yersinia Core-genome Multilocus Sequence Typing for Species Identification and Strain Characterization. *Microbial Genomics* 5(10): e000301. www.microbiologyresearch.org/con tent/journal/mgen/10.1099/mgen.0.000301 [Accessed 24 January 2023].

Schober, S.-M. 2020. Muck, Mummies and Medicine: Disgust in Early Modern Science. *Emotions* 4(1): 43–65.

Secretary, Dept. of Public Health. 1900. Secretary, Dept. of Public Health – Town Clerk. Reconstruction of sewerage at premises 47–51 Sussex. https://

archives.cityofsydney.nsw.gov.au/nodes/view/767441 [Accessed 14 January 2022].

Simmonds, A. 2019. Sex Smells: Olfaction, Modernity and the Regulation of Women's Bodies 1880–1940 (Or How Women Came to Fear Their Own Smells). *Australian Feminist Studies* 34(100): 232–47.

Simond, M., Godley, M. L., & Mouriquand, P. D. E. 1998. Paul-Louis Simond and His Discovery of Plague Transmission by Rat Fleas: A Centenary. *Journal of the Royal Society of Medicine* 91(2): 101–4. https://doi.org/ 10.1177/014107689809100219 [Accessed 19 October 2021].

Simond, P. L., & Yersin, A. 1900. Les épidémies de peste en Extrême-Orient. In *XIIIe Congrès International de Médecine*, 1–60. Paris. https://hal-pasteur .archives-ouvertes.fr/pasteur-00442144 [Accessed 19 October 2021].

Smith, M. M. 2018a. Editor's Introduction: Smelling the Past. In M. M. Smith (ed.), *Smell and History: A Reader*, ix–xxiv. Morgantown: West Virginia University Press

Smith, M. M. 2018b. Making 'Others' Smell. In M. M. Smith (ed.), *Smell and History: A Reader*, 187–201. Morgantown: West Virginia University Press.

Solomon, R. C. 2003. *Not Passion's Slave: Emotions and Choice*. New York: Oxford University Press.

Sunday Times. 1900a. Clergymen at Quarantine Ground. *Sunday Times*. http:// nla.gov.au/nla.news-article126288067 [Accessed 19 November 2021].

Sunday Times. 1900b. Here and There. *Sunday Times*. http://nla.gov.au/nla .news-article126287918 [Accessed 30 January 2023].

Sunday Times. 1900c. Pyrmont's Risks Added To. *Sunday Times*. http://nla.gov .au/nla.news-article126287922 [Accessed 15 January 2022].

Sunday Times. 1900d. The Plague and Lending Libraries. *Sunday Times*. http:// nla.gov.au/nla.news-article126279777 [Accessed 22 October 2021].

Sydney Morning Herald. 1900a. The Bubonic Plague. No Further Developments. *Sydney Morning Herald*. http://nla.gov.au/nla.news-art icle14296543 [Accessed 10 December 2021].

Sydney Morning Herald. 1900b. To the Editor of the Herald. *Sydney Morning Herald*, 8. http://nla.gov.au/nla.news-article14298003 [Accessed 30 January 2023].

Sydney Morning Herald. 1900c. The Bubonic Plague. Discovery of Three More Cases. *Sydney Morning Herald*. http://nla.gov.au/nla.news-article14298675 [Accessed 22 October 2021].

Sydney Morning Herald. 1900d. The Bubonic Plague. Another Household Isolated. *Sydney Morning Herald*. http://nla.gov.au/nla.news-article14299528 [Accessed 24 October 2022].

Sydney Morning Herald. 1900e. The influence in the Western Suburbs. *Sydney Morning Herald*, 10. http://nla.gov.au/nla.news-article28247114 [Accessed 30 January 2023].

Sydney Morning Herald. 1900f. The Bubonic Plague. A Clean Sheet. *Sydney Morning Herald*. http://nla.gov.au/nla.news-article14306853 [Accessed 10 December 2021].

Sydney Morning Herald. 1900g. Chinese Dwellings at Botany. *Sydney Morning Herald*. http://nla.gov.au/nla.news-article14307324 [Accessed 22 October 2021].

Sydney Morning Herald. 1900h. The Bubonic Plague. Cases and Deaths for Two Days. *Sydney Morning Herald*. http://nla.gov.au/nla.news-article14307326 [Accessed 22 October 2021].

Sydney Morning Herald. 1900i. Citizen's Vigilance Committee and the Plague. *Sydney Morning Herald*. http://nla.gov.au/nla.news-article14310239 [Accessed 22 October 2021].

Sydney Morning Herald. 1900j. Citizen's Vigilance Committee. *Sydney Morning Herald*. http://nla.gov.au/nla.news-article14317221 [Accessed 22 October 2021].

Sydney Morning Herald. 1901. Sanitation of the City. *Sydney Morning Herald*. http://nla.gov.au/nla.news-article14415948 [Accessed 15 January 2022].

The Bulletin. 1900a. Vol. 21 No. 1049 (24 March 1900). *The Bulletin*. https://nla.gov.au/nla.obj-661986628 [Accessed 19 November 2021].

The Bulletin. 1900b. Vol. 21 No. 1050 (31 March 1900). *The Bulletin*. https://nla.gov.au/nla.obj-661986644 [Accessed 19 November 2021].

The Bulletin. 1900c. Vol. 21 No. 1053 (21 April 1900). *The Bulletin*. https://nla.gov.au/nla.obj-661986703 [Accessed 19 November 2021].

The Truth. 1900a. Sydney's Baneful Bubo. *The Truth: The People's Paper*. http://nla.gov.au/nla.news-article168000437 [Accessed 19 November 2021].

The Truth. 1900b. The Bubonic 'Black Death'. *The Truth*. http://nla.gov.au/nla.news-article168005840 [Accessed 19 November 2021].

Thearle, J., Jeffs, D., & Heagney, B. 1994. *Plague Revisited: The Black Death: An Account of Plague in Australia, 1900–1923: Prepared for the RACP Annual Scientific Meeting, Hobart May 1994* Rev. ed. Sydney: Royal Australasian College of Physicians.

Tomkins, S. S. 1962. *Affect, Imagery, Consciousness*. New York: Springer.

Town Clerk's Correspondence Folders. 17 July 1900a. Inspector of Nuisances. [Insanitary State of Premises Nos 1, 2 & 3 Washington Lane; Nos 33–37. https://archives.cityofsydney.nsw.gov.au/nodes/view/775514 [Accessed 15 January 2022].

Town Clerk's Correspondence Folders. 25 July 1900b. City Surveyor. Letter to Town Clerk Re Rubbish Carts Tipping on Sand Covering at Moore Park. https://archives.cityofsydney.nsw.gov.au/nodes/view/775363 [Accessed 15 January 2022].

Town Clerk's Correspondence Folders. 26 July 1900c. Citizen's Vigilance Committee – Town Clerk. Filthy state of Belmore markets. Requires Daily. https://archives.cityofsydney.nsw.gov.au/nodes/view/775418 [Accessed 15 January 2022].

Town Clerk's Correspondence Folders. 27 July 1900d. Citizen's Vigilance Committee – Town Clerk. Condition of Premises at 191 Elizabeth St, rats at. https://archives.cityofsydney.nsw.gov.au/nodes/view/775711 [Accessed 15 January 2022].

Turner, V. W. 1967. *The Forest of Symbols: Aspects of Ndembu Ritual [by Victor Turner]*. Ithaca: Cornell University Press.

Tybur, J. M., Molho, C., & Balliet, D. 2020. Moralized Disgust versus Disgusting Immorality: An Adaptationist Perspective. In N. Strohminger & Kumar, Victor (eds.), *The Moral Psychology of Disgust*, 11–25. London: Rowman & Littlefield International.

Waldby, C. 1996. *AIDS and the Body Politic: Biomedicine and Sexual Difference*. London: Routledge.

Watts, S. J. 1997. *Epidemics and History: Disease, Power, and Imperialism*. New Haven: Yale University Press.

Yersin, A., & Treille, G.-F. 1894. La peste bubonique à Hong Kong. In 310–311. *Budapest, Hungary: VIIIe Congres international d'hygiene et de demographie*. https://hal-pasteur.archives-ouvertes.fr/pasteur-00442093 [Accessed 19 October 2021].

Cambridge Elements ≡

Histories of Emotions and the Senses

Series Editors

Rob Boddice
Tampere University

Rob Boddice (PhD, FRHistS) is Senior Research Fellow at the Academy of Finland Centre of Excellence in the History of Experiences. He is the author/editor of 13 books, including *Knowing Pain: A History of Sensation, Emotion and Experience* (Polity Press, 2023), *Humane Professions: The Defence of Experimental Medicine, 1876–1914* (Cambridge University Press, 2021) and *A History of Feelings* (Reaktion, 2019).

Piroska Nagy
Université du Québec à Montréal (UQAM)

Piroska Nagy is Professor of Medieval History at the Université du Québec à Montréal (UQAM) and initiated the first research program in French on the history of emotions. She is the author or editor of 14 volumes, including *Le Don des larmes au Moyen Âge* (Albin Michel, 2000); *Medieval Sensibilities: A History of Emotions in the Middle Ages*, with Damien Boquet (Polity, 2018); and *Histoire des émotions collectives: Épistémologie, émergences, expériences*, with D. Boquet and L. Zanetti Domingues (Classiques Garnier, 2022).

Mark Smith
University of South Carolina

Mark Smith (PhD, FRHistS) is Carolina Distinguished Professor of History and Director of the Institute for Southern Studies at the University of South Carolina. He is author or editor of over a dozen books and his work has been translated into Chinese, Korean, Danish, German, and Spanish. He has lectured in Europe, throughout the United States, Australia, and China and his work has been featured in the New York Times, the London Times, the Washington Post, and the Wall Street Journal. He serves on the US Commission for Civil Rights.

About the Series

Born of the emotional and sensory "turns," Elements in Histories of Emotions and the Senses move one of the fastest-growing interdisciplinary fields forward. The series is aimed at scholars across the humanities, social sciences, and life sciences, embracing insights from a diverse range of disciplines, from neuroscience to art history and economics. Chronologically and regionally broad, encompassing global, transnational, and deep history, it concerns such topics as affect theory, intersensoriality, embodiment, human-animal relations, and distributed cognition. The founding editor of the series was Jan Plamper.

Cambridge Elements ☰

Histories of Emotions and the Senses

Elements in the Series

A full series listing is available at: www.cambridge.org/EHES